HEALTH ADVOCACY

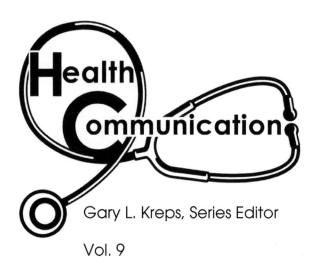

Gary L. Kreps, Series Editor

Vol. 9

The Health Communication series is part of
the Peter Lang Media and Communication list.
Every volume is peer reviewed and meets
the highest quality standards for content and production.

PETER LANG
New York • Bern • Frankfurt • Berlin
Brussels • Vienna • Oxford • Warsaw

MARIFRAN MATTSON & CHERVIN LAM

HEALTH ADVOCACY

A Communication Approach

PETER LANG
New York • Bern • Frankfurt • Berlin
Brussels • Vienna • Oxford • Warsaw

Library of Congress Cataloging-in-Publication Data
Mattson, Marifran, author.
Health advocacy: a communication approach / Marifran Mattson, Chervin Lam.
p. cm. — (Health communication; vol. 9)
Includes bibliographical references and index.
[DNLM: 1. Health Communication—methods. 2. Patient Advocacy.
3. Health Planning—methods. 4. Marketing of Health Services—methods. WA 590]
I. Lam, Chervin, author. II. Title.
III. Series: Health communication (New York, N.Y.); v. 9.
RA427.8   362.1—dc23   2015025399
ISBN 978-1-4331-2423-5 (hardcover)
ISBN 978-1-4539-1714-5 (e-book)
ISSN 2153-1277

Bibliographic information published by **Die Deutsche Nationalbibliothek**.
Die Deutsche Nationalbibliothek lists this publication in the "Deutsche
Nationalbibliografie"; detailed bibliographic data are available
on the Internet at http://dnb.d-nb.de/.

The paper in this book meets the guidelines for permanence and durability
of the Committee on Production Guidelines for Book Longevity
of the Council of Library Resources.

© 2016 Peter Lang Publishing, Inc., New York
29 Broadway, 18th floor, New York, NY 10006
www.peterlang.com

Printed in Germany

DEDICATIONS

To Jim and Simon (woof!), my two strongest and most committed advocates!—MfM

To Jesus Christ, Thomas, and Doris—CL

TABLE OF CONTENTS

ACKNOWLEDGMENTS

Marifran appreciates her Mom, Berni, and Dad, John, for instilling in her the desire and responsibility to serve others, especially those less fortunate. She also acknowledges all those she learned the motivation for and the skills of campaigning from, including her fellow amputees and her professors and mentors. She also recognizes and greatly appreciates Chervin's enthusiasm for and engagement with this book project. Without his effort, this project would still be in process.

Chervin wishes to thank Jesus Christ for the opportunity of graduate school, for helping him throughout this entire book project, and for giving him the strength and ability to write for prolonged hours over many months. Chervin also wishes to thank his parents, Thomas and Doris, for their love and support. Lastly, Chervin wishes to thank Professor Mattson for allowing him to co-author this book; although it was a tiring experience, it also was thoroughly enjoyable and rewarding.

· 1 ·

INTRODUCTION

It was October 4th, a beautiful fall day. The leaves were ablaze in yellow and orange and the sun warmed my cheeks as I admired the scenery. "It's a perfect day!" I thought, as I rode my motorcycle with a few friends. It was a picture-perfect day. I was smiling and relatively relaxed; it was blissful. And then it happened. A truck appeared before me. My mind recognized danger, and a flurry of warning signals hit my senses. I had to dodge, but I knew it was too late—the truck was already too close to me. All I could do was scream.

I knew something bad had happened. I lay motionless on the road and looked up at the perfect blue sky, but its beauty eluded me. There was a deafening silence, an eerie gloom that engulfed me. My friends soon surrounded me, and their expressions confirmed that something serious had occurred. I thought to myself, "Well, I'll let them take care of things here. Maybe I'll just close my eyes and go to sleep." But the idea that I might never wake up suddenly seized me. I was afraid. That pretty fall day turned hostilely cold.

It felt like eons before help arrived. A nurse appeared over my right shoulder, and she said "good that y'all used a tourniquet...but it isn't going to be strong enough." I knew what a tourniquet is. A tool to prevent blood loss. I suppose someone fitted that on me, but I wasn't sure. I couldn't feel pain or comprehend fully the predicament I was in. Someone suggested using a crowbar as reinforcement and then, having found one, wedged it beside my leg. Suddenly a sharp, disturbing pain seized my whole body, and I yelled out in agony. The pain was so piercing it almost caused me to lose consciousness. Soon thereafter my mind finally grasped what had happened to me. My leg was severed.

During this encounter, Professor Mattson lost two-thirds of her blood and, after briefly visiting a hospital emergency reception and talking with her husband, she was rushed via helicopter to a trauma center. The impact with the truck resulted in the amputation of her leg, and she acquired a prosthetic leg months later. After this accident that changed her life, she began to witness problems within the prosthetic community that she never knew existed. Soon, she led an advocacy movement that addressed those problems. She led a legislative effort that resulted in bill HB1140 being passed and signed into law. For amputees in Indiana, this law grants fair access to health insurance coverage for prosthetics (Mattson, 2010). Some of the content in this book explains and illustrates this concept of championing for policy change that impacts the health concerns of specific populations. This notion is known as health advocacy.

Before expounding on health advocacy, it is necessary first to understand some background information and basic definitions that will lead to a more comprehensive appreciation of what health advocacy is. This information includes a brief history of Health Communication, definitions of health, Communication, Health Communication, and health advocacy. Lastly, the Health Communication Advocacy Model will be explained, followed by an exemplar of a health advocacy initiative for illustration.

Abridged History of Health Communication

Communication as an academic discipline has quite a history and many progressive episodes. Its inception often is attributed to Shannon and Weaver's *Mathematical Theory of Communication*, which was developed during the inimical years of the Second World War (Fiske, 2002). Since then, the discipline has proliferated, and its expansion reaches into a variety of areas of interaction such as mass media, organizations, interpersonal relationships, rhetoric, and many more. Extending from the tree of this discipline is *Health Communication*. This branch is a relatively recent and burgeoning area of study; the Health Communication Division of the International Communication Association was founded in 1975. Prior to 1975, research in Health Communication was sporadic, but ever since the field has grown exponentially (Thompson, 2003). However, this growth is not merely expansion, rather it is productive advancement. The field of Health Communication also has been a significant contributor to forwarding academia, with journals such as *Health Communication* making a consistent and significant impact on the social sciences, including disciplines outside of Communication (Feeley, Smith, Moon, & Anker, 2010).

With the size and continuous growth of the field, one might expect scholars to have already reached consensus regarding the definition of Health Communication. Yet, the term still is somewhat obfuscated. Scholars have debated about precise definitions of concepts within the discipline of Communication (Andersen, 1991; Popoff, 2006). Thus, in order to engage in meaningful discourse and study, a conclusive definition of Health Communication has to be established. To achieve this, a perusal of the terms *Health* and *Communication* is required. By ascertaining what these two concepts mean, the notion of Health Communication can be better understood.

Defining Health

When discussing the term *health*, many refer to the World Health Organization (WHO) for its definition, which asserts that "health is a state of complete physical, mental, and social well-being and not merely the absence of disease or infirmity" (2006, p. 1). This definition has been preserved since 1948, but increasingly is met with criticism (Jadad & O'Grady, 2008). One critique is that the idea of being *complete* is far-fetched and impractical. To be absolutely free of any undesirable condition is a lofty goal especially when taking into account the surge in chronic illnesses (Dans et al., 2011; Hamer & El Nahas, 2006; Strong, Mathers, Leeder, & Beaglehole, 2005). Furthermore, the concept of *complete* is dauntingly remote and would label most individuals as ill (Huber et al., 2011). Taking this into account, Huber and colleagues (2011) proposed that instead *health* should be considered "the ability to adapt and to self-manage" (p. 3). That is, to be able to cope independently.

However, the term "independently" should be carefully considered. For example, a person with a disability may be considered independent and self-managing if he or she can make and carry out decisions in the routines of everyday life. This means that requesting and achieving assistance (e.g., assistance into a wheelchair) is a form of independency because the person with a disability had a choice in the matter—from whom he or she requested assistance, the time to assist, the manner it should be performed, and so on. Therefore, independence does not necessarily mean accomplishing everything single-handedly. Rather, independence involves having the autonomy to decide how life tasks should be accomplished. Furthermore, in relation to health, it would be ludicrous to deem someone with a disability as unhealthy, when he or she is independent and is not suffering from virus or disease (Brisenden, 1986).

It also is essential to understand the components that comprise *health*. Bircher (2005) suggested that components of health include psychological, physical, and social aspects. The WHO defined mental health as "a state of well-being in which the individual realizes his or her own abilities, can cope with the normal stresses of life, can work productively and fruitfully, and is able to make a contribution to his or her community" (Herrman, Saxena, & Moodie, 2005, p. 23). Physical wellbeing, on the other hand, is the retention of physiological equilibrium in the face of a malignant environment (Huber et al., 2011). As for social health, Russell (as cited in McDowell, 2006) suggested that it is "that dimension of an individual's well-being that concerns how he gets along with other people, how other people react to him, and how he interacts with social institutions and societal mores" (p. 150). These three elements—psychological, physical, and social states—holistically represent the concept of *health*.

Taking into consideration the aforementioned concepts, we forward the following definition of health:

> Health is the ability to cope independently in opposition to forces that disorientate the psychological, physical, or social equilibrium by staying oriented to or realigning to that equilibrium.

Defining Communication

Communication, in its barest and simplest form, is the "process of understanding and sharing meaning" (Pearson & Nelson, 2000, p. 3). This definition suggests that communication occurs copiously everywhere in everyday life. It is present in daily human interactions, organizations, mass media, and in any form of medium (see Akkirman & Harris, 2005; Chen & Huang, 2007; McQuail, 2010). Most often communication involves primarily two parties—a sender of a message and a receiver of the message. In a scenario where congruent interaction is desired, the former should have clarity and succinctness in delivering a message, while the latter should pay attention and have effective and coherent decoding of the message (Dewatripont, & Tirole, 2005). The message can be verbal and nonverbal—the former being the spoken word and the latter being symbols not represented by language, including gestures, appearance, vocal cues, eye movements, and so on (Knapp, 2012). It is difficult to establish whether these are intentional or unintentional, and there is ongoing debate among scholars over the two perspectives (Andersen, 1991; Motley, 1986). However, most scholars agree that communication occurs only when there is a receiver who takes in the message. Without the recipient of the message, there is no communication (Andersen, 1991). Based on the need for a receiver, communication would only occur if there are two or more individuals. Mattson and Hall (2011) echoed this by highlighting that communication is a transactional process (p. 22), which involves a sender of a message, a recipient, and an avenue for feedback. Although there may be instances where communication is somewhat one-sided (e.g., radio, television), most communication occurs within transactional situations.

Thus, taking all this into account, we offer the following definition of communication:

> Communication is a verbal and nonverbal transaction where a message is generated by a sender and received and interpreted by a receiver who provides feedback in an effort to achieve mutual understanding.

Defining Health Communication

Now that the terms *health* and *communication* have been respectively elucidated, it is necessary to integrate the two into one single concept: Health Communication. In order to achieve a comprehensive definition, it also is imperative to examine the objective of this discipline and discover how it is distinct from other forms of Communication Studies.

A key goal of Health Communication is to impact people and communities for the betterment of their health (Schiavo, 2007). For example, a $48 million public health communication campaign in Thailand influenced the decline in new HIV infections from 143,000 in the year 1991 to 29,000 in 2000. This included large communicative efforts as 488 radio stations and 15 television stations were utilized to air HIV/AIDS prevention messages each hour (Singhal & Rogers, 2003). Evidently, such public health communication campaigns have impactful and positive outcomes. The ability to fuse academic findings with practical action can result in huge benefits for society, and there is a need for more scholars to be involved and to engage in greater collaboration with field practitioners (Babrow & Mattson, 2003; Clift, 1997; Nzyuko, 1996). This notion of applying theory to service action is congruent with the service-learning approach, during which learning and engagement intersect. Such a method is increasingly popular in academia, and it is potentially beneficial for academics to adopt because skills and knowledge may be enhanced from community service involvement. There has been incremental use of the service-learning method, and students have experienced the heightening of multicultural awareness through such application (Oster-Aaland, Sellnow, Nelson, & Pearson, 2004). Engaging with people in action is thus a mutually advantageous responsibility that academics, students, and communities can thrive from. Therefore, a crucial aspect of Health Communication is to serve or engage people in improving health concerns.

Health Communication is a branch of Communication Studies, legitimate and distinct from its sibling subfields such as interpersonal communication, mass communication, and organizational communication. There were criticisms surrounding this claim of distinctiveness, but increasingly, it is clearer how Health Communication is truly unique (Nussbaum, 1989). Although there may be instances of interpersonal or media communication processes mentioned in its literature, the settings, agenda, and focus are so markedly different that it has become a field of its own. Also, there are a lot of interpersonal, media, and psychological elements in Health Communication (Ratzan, 1996), but if scholars refuse to accept it as a distinct field, a problem arises in that academics would never agree on which field it should be subsumed under—interpersonal communication, media studies, or psychology. The reason there can be no consensus is because all three are prominently used. The word "used" is stressed because theories and ideas are plucked from these other disciplines as tools to build an academic arena, in this case Health Communication. The utilization of various disciplines is ultimately for the purposes of construction, not imitation.

For instance, a good amount of studies in Health Communication examine patient and healthcare provider interaction, and these studies utilize concepts found in interpersonal, socioeconomic, and social identity studies (Jensen, King, Guntzviller, & Davis, 2010; Johnson, Roter, Powe, & Cooper, 2004; Roter, 1977). To suggest that a study of patient-healthcare provider interaction is merely a branch of interpersonal communication would be remiss by not considering socioeconomic and social identity literatures. Furthermore, it would neither be fair nor reasonable for any of these subfields to claim possession of the patient-healthcare provider subject, for each is used only occasionally, when relevant or appropriate. Thus, it is essential that Health Communication be a field in its own right so that research such as patient-healthcare provider interaction has an academic and practical place to consider home within the discipline of Communication.

Due to the interdisciplinary nature of Health Communication, it may be more useful to understand it in terms of the themes often studied. Health Communication revolves around assessment of health-related concerns, and the themes oftentimes include evaluations of risk (see e.g., Cho & Witte, 2005; Rosenstock, Strecher, & Becker, 1988), decision-making processes (see e.g., Afifi & Steuber, 2009; Ajzen, 1991; Sheppard, Hartwick, & Warshaw, 1988; Yang, McComas, Gay, Leonard, Dannenberg, & Dillon, 2010), uncertainty management (see e.g., Babrow, 2001; Brashers, 2001; Kramer, 1999), analysis of health disparities (see e.g., Braveman, 2006; Gordon-Larsen, Nelson, Page, & Popkin, 2006), patient-healthcare provider interaction (see e.g., Cooper-Patrick, Gallo, Gonzales, Vu, Powe, Nelson, & Ford, 1999), health campaigns (see e.g., Snyder, 2007), and health advocacy (Mindell, Sheridan, Joffe, Samson-Barry, & Atkinson, 2004). The common thread that ties these themes together is that they all involve communication processes. Much of the research that Health Communication scholars embark upon emphasizes understanding and application of communication processes within health-related issues.

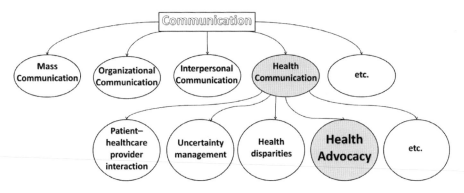

Figure 1.1: Subfields in Communication.

Tying all these threads together then, we define the term Health Communication as:

> The study and/or practice of communication that aims to address health issues/concerns by considering the communication processes involved.

Defining Health Advocacy

In the broad spectrum of Health Communication, there is a growing emphasis in the discipline to engage with individuals and communities, to help alleviate concerns surrounding health through communication strategies, and to further reinforce the processes that already inspire and maintain people's health. This engagement on behalf of individual and community health is the basis of *health advocacy*. To advocate for health is to be a proponent for change—a change for both industry and authorities to alter decisions that influence the health choices people make, to influence public policy and prompt for regulation, and to spur change in systems to benefit people's health (Lupton, 1994). The American Public Health Association (APHA, 2002) adds that advocacy can educate the public and change public opinion, too.

There are a few methods for advocacy. One common tool is the use of media, which can assist in amplifying a community's concerns, legitimize its cause, and lend strength to its goals (Wallack & Dorfman, 1996). The use of media can lead to widespread dissemination of information, and is therefore highly useful for promoting campaigns and for building awareness. To be sure, media are not the only mechanisms that can be utilized for advocacy. Another approach involves forming lobbying groups, which may help emancipate people from hegemonic oppression, thus allowing them to strive for change in policies (Lupton, 1994).

Advocacy is about championing a cause. It involves instigating change for people whose lives are marginalized or in need of improvement. For instance, in 2004, the National African American Tobacco Prevention Network collaborated to vanquish Kool, a flavored cigarette that targeted African American youth. The network successfully abolished Kool and was awarded $1.4 million in settlement. This victory was reminiscent of another success in the 1990s, when Stop Uptown Cigarettes brought an end to Uptown Cigarettes, which also targeted African Americans (Freudenberg, Bradley, & Serrano, 2009). Thus, advocacy is about leading change.

It is vital to juxtapose the terms *health advocacy* and *advocacy*, because they correspond, yet are different. The former is concerned with championing causes directly related to health matters, and the latter is more generic, and encompasses causes on all types of issues. An illustrative example of health advocacy is the Indiana Amputee Insurance Protection Coalition's engagement with the amputee community and related organizations within Indiana to pursue greater access to prosthetic devices. Their efforts were successful—a bill, HB1140, was passed and signed into law, which granted prosthetic parity across health insurance plans in Indiana. This allowed many amputees to acquire prosthetic limbs which otherwise would have been difficult, if not impossible, to obtain (Mattson, 2010). For an example of advocacy that is not directly related to health issues, consider the Association of Community Organizations for Reform Now, which advocates for low-income families. They launched a movement against Edison Schools to address the management of low-performing schools in New York and Philadelphia (Scott, Lubienski, & DeBray-Pelot, 2009). Granted, the latter example is admirable and good for society, but it does not pertain directly to health concerns, and therefore is not the subject focus of this book. Rather, what is delved into within this book is advocacy for health-related issues. With this explanation, and for simplicity's sake, this book will use the terms *health advocacy* and *advocacy* interchangeably with the understanding that the context of advocacy is health related.

As a final definitional consideration, there needs to be clarification about how health advocacy from a communication perspective differs from public health advocacy (see e.g., Christoffel, 2000). Both perspectives and the approaches associated with them are invested in improving health through advocacy, but as communication scholars, we are interested in the *communication processes* involved in advocacy efforts. For instance, health advocacy research from a communication perspective might consider the interactions within a grassroots organization, the communication theories in campaign and media strategies, the interpersonal relationships forged and contested in networks and rallies, and so on. As communication scholars, we distinguish ourselves in that our focus is on the communication processes and theories involved in health advocacy, as well as the resulting outcomes from health communication advocacy efforts. For this reason, it is fitting and correct to infer that *health advocacy* in this context can also mean *health communication advocacy*; so these terms may be used interchangeably. For the sake of simplicity though, the term *advocacy* in this book refers to the same concept as *health communication advocacy*. The important point to remember is that health advocacy from a communication perspective has a primary focus on communication processes involved in advocacy.

Given all these considerations, we coin the following definition of health advocacy:

> Health advocacy is the attempted effort to change health policies so that better health outcomes may result.

Health Communication Advocacy Model

The *Health Communication Advocacy Model* (Mattson, 2010) is an extension of the message development tool for health campaigns (Mattson & Basu, 2010a, 2010b) and the social marketing framework (Kotler & Lee, 2008). This model emphasizes the message design process, particularly in the tailoring of messages to address needs of the audience. The model is a framework that attempts to allow users of the model to execute and go through an advocacy effort for any health issue in an efficient and effective manner. Thus, its application is not limited to a few health issues, but can be utilized for various health concerns such as issues in obesity, cancer, smoking, and so forth. There are three phases in the Health Communication Advocacy Model.

In the first phase, an advocacy team is assembled, and its size can range from a small group, to a moderate sized committee, or a large coalition. The team should consist of a health issue expert, community partners, public health/communication specialists, and possibly a lobbyist, if the advocacy effort has a political reach. During this phase, members discuss basic but important matters such as individual roles and responsibilities, approaches and strategies for fund-raising, whether or not to hire a lobbyist, and—most importantly—their position statement on the health issue they are advocating for. After these tasks accomplished, the team can transition to Phase 2.

In Phase 2, strategic planning from formative research is conducted. The team will determine the prevailing advocacy needs of the target population affected by the health issue, which may be derived through research and statistical records. The team also will identify who are the legislators, relevant populations, and media for message dissemination. Once the needs assessment is conducted, tailored advocacy messages will be developed using communication theories. To the extent possible, draft messages should be pretested with the target audiences to obtain feedback for improving the messages. Once the team is confident in the effectiveness of drafted messages, they can proceed to Phase 3.

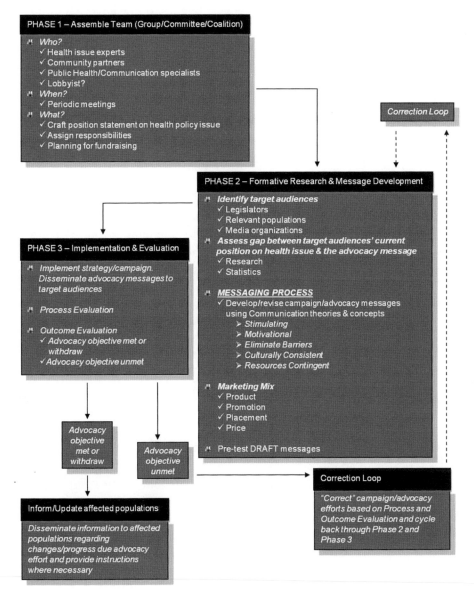

Figure 1.2: Health Communication Advocacy Model.

Phase 3 involves implementation of strategies and evaluation of the team's efforts and outcome. In this phase the team executes their strategies of disseminating advocacy messages to the target audiences, such as rallying, attending legislative committee meetings, providing testimony through media, and so on. Throughout this process the effectiveness of the advocacy effort is monitored by tracking the strategy, such as the number of media hits, legislative votes, and signatures for the team's petition. The outcome evaluation is the assessment of the end result, for instance, whether votes in the Senate and House favored the team's position statement on the health issue. If the objective is not met, the team would proceed to the Correction Loop phase.

In the Correction Loop, the evaluations of the process and outcome are analyzed, and the team uses the lessons learned from the analysis to further improve their campaign efforts. The team may need to return to Phase 2, where there is a reassessment of needs and revised messages are developed. This Correction Loop continues until the team decides to withdraw or the team considers that they have met their advocacy objective.

Based on this understanding of the Health Communication Advocacy Model, an exemplar is presented to illustrate the application of this model and the effectiveness of advocacy initiatives that adhere to this model.

An Exemplar of a Health Advocacy Initiative

After the events described in the opening of this chapter, Professor Mattson was fitted with a C-leg—an advanced prosthetic that has a computerized knee and a stumble-recovery system. The cost for this prosthetic was daunting—more than $50,000. Initially the health insurance company was reluctant to pay for the costs and deemed such an advanced prosthetic unnecessary. Professor Mattson filed a dispute, and through arguments that she needed a C-leg for independent living including the ability to work, the insurance company eventually helped pay for it. This grueling episode was resolved because of her training in debate, persuasion, and Health Communication, which left her to wonder—what if she wasn't equipped with such skills? Would she have to settle for a prosthetic leg with less functionality or, worse, be left to function without a prosthetic at all?

Later, she discovered that many of the almost 2 million amputees in the United States were living without prosthetics because their health insurance plans stopped covering prosthetics or because their coverage was insufficient to help pay for a prosthetic. This situation was puzzling to her because she believed that people should be covered by their health insurance for catastrophic illness or injuries since they had paid premiums for insurance. Eventually, Professor Mattson was asked to lead an advocacy initiative to pass prosthetic parity legislation in Indiana. Such legislation would require commercial health insurance carriers to provide coverage for the purchasing, replacing, and repairing of prosthetic devices and components. After hearing the benefits it would bring for prosthetically-challenged amputees, she agreed to lead the advocacy effort. To inform the effort, Professor Mattson made revisions to the message development tool for health campaigns that she was working on with Ambar Basu (Mattson & Basu, 2010a, 2010b) so that it would be applicable to an advocacy campaign, and her team adhered to the model in their advocacy efforts.

For Phase 1, the team formed the Indiana Amputee Insurance Protection Coalition, which was comprised of amputees, caregivers, prosthetic manufacturers and providers, and a Health Communication specialist. They drafted their position statement for the health issue (i.e., prosthetic parity), and brainstormed strategies for fundraising. They also determined that a lobbyist was needed, and they hired a lobbyist who had valuable networks and experience in legislation and in acquiring endorsements from relevant organizations such as the American Diabetes Association and the Indiana Medical Association.

In Phase 2, the team conducted a needs assessment by researching prosthetic parity efforts in other states and estimated that costs for residents of Indiana would be approximately $2 per year per health insurance plan participant. In the messaging process, messages were specifically crafted for and tailored to their target audiences, which included people who would be affected by the legislation (i.e., amputees, caregivers), the legislators, and the media. Statistics and testimonials were to be used to persuade legislators, a prosthetic parity petition was written for amputees and their friends and family to sign, and press releases were designed for the media.

In Phase 3, the team's strategy was implemented as they rallied amputees at the statehouse and presented testimony at legislative committee meetings. The team conducted process evaluation by tracking the number of signatures in favor of their petition prior to submitting it to legislators, monitoring the number of media hits, and tracking the legislative votes in favor of their position. The outcome evaluation was the result of the final vote in the Indiana Senate and House, which garnered 44 to 3 votes in their favor for the former and 72 to 25 for the latter. When the governor signed for the bill to pass, the team accomplished their objective—prosthetic parity across insurance plans became law in Indiana!

Had the team failed to obtain enough votes in their favor, the team would have proceeded to the Correction Loop, where they would reevaluate their efforts, formulate a better strategy, and return to Phase 2 where they would have to plan and design improved messages and dissemination of those messages.

This however, was not necessary for Professor Mattson and her team, as their bill, HB1140, was passed. The testimonies of amputees who benefited from the legislation were encouraging and rewarding. For instance, a 10-year-old double amputee, Evan, finally had insurance coverage for two prosthetic legs when he outgrew his prosthetics. Prior to that, his health insurance carrier would only help pay for one but not two prosthetic legs. Another beneficiary, Harold, finally received a properly fitting prosthetic leg when, prior to the law change, he was told by his health insurance carrier that he had to shed 20 pounds of weight before they would approve a new prosthetic leg.

These are two of the many lives that were impacted by the advocacy efforts which resulted in changes in the law in favor of prosthetic parity. However, the Health Communication Advocacy Model is not limited to championing for prosthetic rights—it can be used for various health-related issues as well. With adherence to and application of this advocacy model, teams should be able to lead an advocacy effort successfully and accomplish its desired advocacy goals.

Summary

Health Communication is a relatively new subfield that focuses on the application of communication theories and concepts to health-related issues. Branching from this is health advocacy, which is the study of communication processes that aim to change systems, policies, beliefs, attitudes, and/or behaviors for the betterment of the health of individuals and communities. Using the Health Communication Advocacy Model, a team can lead a health advocacy effort efficiently and likely achieve its desired advocacy goals. The following chapters in this book examine in greater detail the components of the Health Communication Advocacy Model. The next chapter begins by providing an overview of the meta-theoretical foundation of the Health Communication Advocacy Model—Systems Theory.

References

Afifi, T., & Steuber, K. (2009). The revelation risk model (RRM): Factors that predict the revelation of secrets and the strategies used to reveal them. *Communication Monographs*, 76(2), 144–176. doi: 10.1080/03637750902828412

Ajzen, I. (1991). The theory of planned behavior. *Organizational Behavior and Human Decision Processes*, 50(2), 179–211. doi: 10.1016/0749-5978(91)90020-T

Akkirman, A. D., & Harris, D. L. (2005). Organizational communication satisfaction in the virtual workplace. *Journal of Management Development*, 24(5), 397–409. doi: 10.1108/02621710510598427

American Public Health Association (2002). *APHA media advocacy manual*. Unpublished manuscript, Washington, DC.

Andersen, P. A. (1991). When one cannot not communicate: A challenge to Motley's traditional communication postulates. *Communication Studies*, 42(4), 309–325. doi: 10.1080/10510979109368346

Babrow, A. S. (2001). Uncertainty, value, communication, and problematic integration. *Journal of Communication*, 51(3), 553–573. doi: 10.1111/j.1460-2466.2001.tb02896.x

Babrow, A. S., Mattson, M. (2003). Building health communication theories in the 21st century. In T. L. Thompson, A. M. Dorsey, K. I. Miller, & R. Parrott (Eds.), *Handbook of Health Communication* (pp. 35–61). Mahwah, NJ: Lawrence Erlbaum Associates, Inc.

Bircher, J. (2005). Towards a dynamic definition of health and disease. *Medicine, Health Care and Philosophy*, 8(3), 335–341. doi: 10.1007/s11019-005-0538-y

Brashers, D. E. (2001). Communication and uncertainty management. *Journal of Communication*, 51(3), 477–497. doi: 10.1111/j.1460-2466.2001.tb02892.x

Braveman, P. (2006). Health disparities and health equity: Concepts and measurement. *Annual Review of Public Health*, 27, 167–194. doi: 10.1146/annurev.publhealth.27.021405.102103

Brisenden, S. (1986). Independent living and the medical model of disability. *Disability, Handicap & Society*, 1(2), 173–178. Retrieved from http://www.tandf.co.uk/journals/titles/09687599.aspl

Chen, C. J., & Huang, J. W. (2007). How organizational climate and structure affect knowledge management—The social interaction perspective. *International Journal of Information Management*, 27(2), 104–118. doi:10.1016/j.ijinfomgt.2006.11.001

Cho, H., & Witte, K. (2005). Managing fear in public health campaigns: A theory-based formative evaluation process. *Health Promotion Practice*, 6(4), 482–490. doi: 10.1177/1524839904263912

Christoffel, K. K. (2000). Public health advocacy: Process and product. *American Journal of Public Health*, 90(5), 722. Retrieved from http://www.ajph.org/

Clift, E. (1997). What do you say you do? Health communicators and where we fit in. *Journal of Health Communication*, 2, 65–67. doi: 10.1080/108107397127932

Cooper-Patrick, L., Gallo, J. J., Gonzales, J. J., Vu, H. T., Powe, N. R., Nelson, C., & Ford, D. E. (1999). Race, gender, and partnership in the patient-physician relationship. *JAMA: The Journal of the American Medical Association*, 282(6), 583–589. doi:10.1001/jama.282.6.583.

Dans, A., Ng, N., Varghese, C., Tai, E. S., Firestone, R., & Bonita, R. (2011). The rise of chronic non-communicable diseases in Southeast Asia: Time for action. *The Lancet, 377*(9766), 680–689. doi: 10.1016/S0140–6736(10)61506–1

Dewatripont, M., & Tirole, J. (2005). Modes of communication. *Journal of Political Economy, 113*(6), 1217–1238. Retrieved from http://www.journals.uchicago.edu/

Feeley, T., H., Smith, R., A., Moon, S., & Anker, A., E. (2010). A journal-level analysis of Health Communication. *Health Communication, 25* (6–7), 516–521. doi: 10.1080/10410236.2010.496604

Fiske, J. (2002). *Introduction to communication studies*. New York: Taylor & Francis.

Freudenberg, N., Bradley, S. P., & Serrano, M. (2009). Public health campaigns to change industry practices that damage health: An analysis of 12 case studies. *Health Education & Behavior, 36*(2), 230–249. doi: 10.1177/1090198107301330

Gordon-Larsen, P., Nelson, M. C., Page, P., & Popkin, B. M. (2006). Inequality in the built environment underlies key health disparities in physical activity and obesity. *Pediatrics, 117*(2), 417–424. doi: 10.1542/peds. 2005–0058

Hamer, R. A., & El Nahas, A. M. (2006). The burden of chronic kidney disease: Is rising rapidly worldwide. *BMJ: British Medical Journal, 332*(7541), 563. Retrieved from http://group.bmj.com/

Herrman, H., Saxena, S., & Moodie, R. (2005). *Promoting mental health: Concepts, emerging evidence, practice: A report of the World Health Organization, Department of Mental Health and Substance Abuse in collaboration with the Victorian Health Promotion Foundation and the University of Melbourne*. World Health Organization. Retrieved from http://www.who.int

Huber, M., Knottnerus, J. A., Green, L., Horst, H. V. D., Jadad, A. R., Kromhout, D., ... & Smid, H. (2011). How should we define health? *BMJ: British Medical Journal, 343*, 1–3. doi:10.1136/bmj.d4163

Jadad, A. R., & O'Grady, L. (2008). How should health be defined? *BMJ: British Medical Journal, 337*. doi: 10.1136/bmj.a2900

Jensen, J. D., King, A. J., Guntzviller, L. M., & Davis, L. A. (2010). Patient-provider communication and low-income adults: Age, race, literacy, and optimism predict communication satisfaction. *Patient Education and Counseling, 79*(1), 30–35. doi:10.1016/j.pec.2009.09.041

Johnson, R. L., Roter, D., Powe, N. R., & Cooper, L. A. (2004). Patient race/ethnicity and quality of patient-physician communication during medical visits. *American Journal of Public Health, 94*(12), 2084–2090. Retrieved from http://www.ajph.org/

Kersh, R. (2000). State autonomy & civil society: The lobbyist connection. *Critical Review, 14*(2–3), 237–257. doi: 10.1080/08913810008443559

Knapp, M. L. (2012). *Nonverbal communication in human interaction*. Boston, MA: Cengage Learning.

Kotler, P., & Lee, N. R. (2008). *Social marketing: Influencing behaviors for good* (3rd ed.). Thousand Oaks, CA: Sage.

Kramer, M. W. (1999). Motivation to reduce uncertainty: A reconceptualization of Uncertainty Reduction Theory. *Management Communication Quarterly, 13*(2), 305–316. doi: 10.1177/0893318999132007

Lupton, D. (1994). Toward the development of critical health communication praxis. *Health Communication*, 6(1), 55–67. doi: 10.1207/s15327027hc0601_4

Mattson, M. (2010). Health advocacy by accident and discipline. *Health Communication*, 25(6–7), 622–624. doi: 10.1080/10410236.2010.496844

Mattson, M., & Basu, A. (2010a). Center for Disease Control's diethylstilbestrol update: A case for effective operationalization of messaging in social marketing practice. *Health Promotion Practice*, 11(4), 580–588. doi: 10.1177/1524839908324785

Mattson, M., & Basu, A. (2010b). The message development tool: A case for effective operationalization of messaging in social marketing practice. *Health Marketing Quarterly*, 27(3), 275–290. doi: 10.1080/07359683.2010.495305

Mattson, M., & Hall, J. G. (2011). *Health as communication nexus*. Dubuque, IA: Kendall Hunt.

McDowell, I. (2006). *Measuring health: A guide to rating scales and questionnaires* (3rd ed.). New York, NY: Oxford University Press.

McGrath, C. (2005). *Lobbying in Washington, London, and Brussels: The persuasive communication of political issues*. Lewiston, NY: Edwin Mellen Press.

McGrath, C. (2007). Lobbying and the 2006 U.S. midterm elections. *Journal of Public Affairs*, 7(2), 192–203. doi: 10.1002/pa.257

McQuail, D. (2010). *McQuail's mass communication theory*. Thousand Oaks, CA: Sage Publications.

Mindell, J., Sheridan, L., Joffe, M., Samson-Barry, H., & Atkinson, S. (2004). Health impact assessment as an agent of policy change: Improving the health impacts of the mayor of London's draft transport strategy. *Journal of Epidemiology & Community Health*, 58(3), 169–174. doi: 10.1136/jech.2003.012385

Motley, M. T. (1986). Consciousness and intentionality in communication: A preliminary model and methodological approaches. *Western Journal of Speech Communication*, 50(1), 3–23. doi: 10.1080/10570318609374210

Nussbaum, J. F. (1989). Directions for research within health communication. *Health Communication*, 1(1), 35–40. doi: 10.1207/ s15327027hc0101_5

Nzyuko, S. (1996). Does research have any role in information/education/communication programs in Africa? An insider's view. *Journal of Health Communication*, 1(2), 227–229. doi: 10.1080/108107396128167

Oster-Aaland, L., Sellnow, T. L., Nelson, P. E., & Pearson, J. C. (2004). The status of service learning in departments of communication: A follow-up study. *Communication Education*, 53(4), 348–356. doi: 10.10/0363452032000305959

Pearson, J. C., & Nelson, P. E. (2000). *An introduction to human communication: Understanding and sharing* (8th ed.). Boston, MA: McGraw-Hill.

Popoff, D. (2006). The communication journal collection. *Collection Management*, 30(3), 67–85. doi: 10.1300/J105v30n03_06

Ratzan, S. C. (1996). The status and scope of health communication. *Journal of Health Communication*, 1(1), 25–42. doi: 10.1080/108107396128211

Rosenstock, I. M., Strecher, V. J., & Becker, M. H. (1988). Social learning theory and the health belief model. *Health Education & Behavior*, *15*(2), 175–183. doi: 10.1177/109019818801500203

Roter, D. L. (1977). Patient participation in the patient-provider interaction: The effects of patient question asking on the quality of interaction, satisfaction and compliance. *Health Education & Behavior*, *5*(4), 281–315. doi: 10.1177/109019817700500402

Schiavo, R. (2007). *Health communication: From theory to practice*. San Francisco, CA: Jossey-Bass.

Scott, J., Lubienski, C., & DeBray-Pelot, E. (2009). The politics of advocacy in education. *Educational Policy*, *23*(1), 3–14. doi: 10.1177/0895904808328530

Sheppard, B. H., Hartwick, J., & Warshaw, P. R. (1988). The theory of reasoned action: A meta-analysis of past research with recommendations for modifications and future research. *Journal of Consumer Research*, 325–343. Retrieved from http://ejcr.org

Singhal, A., & Rogers, E. M. (2003). *Combating AIDS: Communication strategies in action*. New Delhi, India: Sage.

Snyder, L. B. (2007). Health communication campaigns and their impact on behavior. *Journal of Nutrition Education and Behavior*, *39*(2), S32–S40. doi: 10.1016/j.jneb.2006.09.004

Strong, K., Mathers, C., Leeder, S., & Beaglehole, R. (2005). Preventing chronic diseases: How many lives can we save? *The Lancet*, *366*(9496), 1578–1582. doi: 10.1016/S0140-6736(05)67341-2

Thomas, C. S., Hrebenar, R. J. (2009). Comparing lobbying across liberal democracies: Problems, approaches and initial findings. *Journal of Comparative Politics*, *2*(1), 131–142. Retrieved from http://www.jofcp.org/jcp/

Thompson, T. L. (2003). Introduction. In T. L. Thompson, A. M. Dorsey, K. I. Miller, & R. Parrott (Eds.), *Handbook of Health Communication* (pp. 1–5). Mahwah, NJ: Lawrence Erlbaum Associates, Inc.

Vidal, J. B. I., Draca, M., & Fons-Rosen, C. (2012). Revolving door lobbyists. *The American Economic Review*, *102*(7), 3731–3748. doi: 10.1257/aer.102.7.3731

Wallack, L., & Dorfman, L. (1996). Media advocacy: A strategy for advancing policy and promoting health. *Health Education & Behavior*, *23*(3), 293–317. doi: 10.1177/109019819602300303

World Health Organization (2006). *Constitution of the World Health Organization Supplement* (pp. 1—18). Retrieved from http://www.who.int

Yang, J. Z., McComas, K., Gay, G., Leonard, J. P., Dannenberg, A. J., & Dillon, H. (2010). From information processing to behavioral intentions: Exploring cancer patients' motivations for clinical trial enrollment. *Patient Education and Counseling*, *79*(2), 231–238. doi: 10.1016/j.pec.2009.08.010

· 2 ·

SYSTEMS THEORY

The Health Communication Advocacy Model is consistent with the principles of systems theory, which posits that a system is complex and relies on interdependent component parts (Miller, 2012). Initially, systems theory was introduced by biologist Ludwig Von Bertalanffy, as a concept that could help explain how a physical system, a plant, operates (Von Bertalanffy, 1968). Although in the social sciences, systems theory typically is applied in organizational contexts (e.g., business operations), this chapter considers how systems theory can be applied to guide how a health advocacy campaign operates as a dynamic system. Specifically, systems theory will be used to explain the properties and mechanisms of the Health Communication Advocacy Model. We begin by explaining what systems theory is and how systems theory is a metatheory. Thereafter, the chapter considers the Health Communication Advocacy Model through the lens of systems theory, including the properties, components, and processes inherent in the model.

Systems Theory as a Metatheory

Metatheory is the analysis and examination of theories (Haas & Mattson, 2015; Zhao, 1991). That is to say, metatheory is a theory of theories. For example, when one examines an existing theory and revises the theory based on empirical findings and/or other theoretical input, metatheorizing would have taken place (see e.g., Mattson, 1999). A metatheory also may involve the combination of theories to develop a new theory or concept. Systems theory is a metatheory in part because ideas from biology were borrowed to formulate a multidisciplinary theory that also could be applied in the social sciences (Miller, 2012).

Systems theory helps describe and explain how systems operate. The theory advances the perspective that, like biological systems, human social systems also are open and interactive as opposed to being closed and in isolation from their environment (Miller, 2012). For example, a systems theory perspective posits that an organization should collaborate with other organizations in order to grow and survive (e.g., open innovation; see Gassmann, Enkel, & Chesbrough, 2010). In that vein, a systems theory perspective for a health advocacy campaign would emphasize the need for the campaign to account for environmental factors in order for the advocacy campaign model or approach to be effective. For example, the advocacy campaign model would need to consider how people may react and how situational changes may affect progression in the campaign. The campaign system or the model on which the campaign is based operates very similarly to that of an organization, such as having its own components.

System Components

Like an organization, a model has components that make up the entire system. An example of the former may be the departments that make up an organization, while an example of the latter may be the phases in a model (i.e., Phase 1, Phase 2, Phase 3, etc.). According to systems theory, components of a system have three characteristics: hierarchical ordering, interdependence, and permeability (Miller, 2012). The components of the Health Communication Advocacy Model also share these characteristics.

Hierarchical ordering refers to the levels that exist among components. Specifically, these levels are subsystems and supersystems (Miller, 2012). Subsystems are parts of a system that have a narrower focus while supersystems have a broader focus. In the context of a model, a subsystem may be a part of the model that addresses a specific concern, while a supersystem may be a part of the model that covers a broad range of concerns. For example, a subsystem in the Health Communication Advocacy Model may be the Messaging Process stage, where messages are developed (see Chapter 6). A supersystem for the Health Communication Advocacy Model may be the Formative Research and Message Development Phase, which encompasses the Messaging Process *and* the Needs Assessment and Marketing Mix stages (see Figure 2.1).

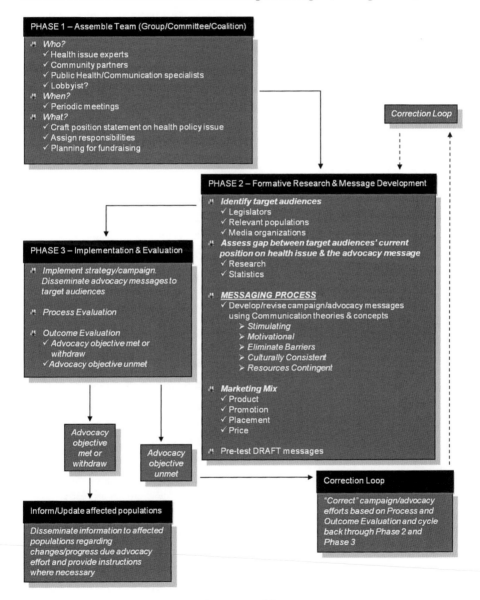

Figure 2.1: Health Communication Advocacy Model.

To take the characteristic of hierarchical ordering even further, the "stimulating" category in the Messaging Process stage may be considered as a smaller subsystem. It is essential to note that hierarchical ordering does not mean that subsystems are less important than supersystems. Instead, subsystems and supersystems are descriptors and each is a vital component of a model that is required for the model to operate and be effective. That is to say that subsystems and supersystems are mutually important or interdependent.

According to systems theory, components in a system are interdependent. In the context of the Health Communication Advocacy Model, this means that each phase in the model requires the other phases in the model in order to work and be effective. For example, Phase 3 of the Health Communication Advocacy Model only can begin after Phase 2 is completed; disseminating messages can only take place after research is conducted and messages are developed. By the same token, Phase 2 relies on Phase 3 in order to be useful; without implementation of advocacy messages during Phase 3, the development of advocacy messages in Phase 2 would be for naught. Thus, the phases or components of the model are interdependent.

Systems theory also posits that components of a system need to be permeable. Components are permeable if they are open to environmental factors, which may include interactions with or responses from audiences and situational changes. The phases (i.e., components) of the Health Communication Advocacy Model are permeable because they account for these environmental factors. For example, in Phase 2, the Pre-Test Draft Message stage, the model considers audiences' receptivity to draft advocacy messages and recommends refining advocacy messages accordingly. In a closed system, the components of the model are *not* permeable and in the example of advocacy, the team would not take into account feedback from audiences but instead would insist on forwarding its own communication strategy. The Health Communication Advocacy Model also considers situational changes. For example, the Assemble Team Phase (i.e., Phase 1) is not rigid and allows for situational changes. For instance, if the advocacy team runs into a situation during which the budget becomes limited, the team may attempt advocacy without a lobbyist, although a lobbyist is recommended. In contrast, an advocacy model with impermeable components would not be concerned about situational changes and would insist on progressing through the model regardless of changes in the environment. However, given that audience feedback is important and that situational circumstances may arise, it is imperative for the Health Communication Advocacy Model to have permeable components so that the model can adapt to change.

System Processes

A system that has permeable components must take into consideration environmental interactions in its processes. A model with open or permeable components will operate assuming that the environment will significantly influence and shape its processes, including during input, throughput, and output processes (Miller, 2012).

Input refers to the transactional process during which information is taken from the environment and entered into the system. In the context of the Health Communication Advocacy Model, for example, the input process occurs when formative research about the advocated health issue is conducted. During this process, information regarding the advocated health issue, such as statistical evidence about the health issue, is taken into the system and used for developing and disseminating relevant and effective advocacy messages. This message development and dissemination process is known as the throughput process, during which input information is used to generate an output. The output process involves generating a product from the system. In the context of the Health Communication Advocacy Model, an output would refer to the advocacy outcome. That is, whether or not the advocacy messages were successful in bringing about health policy change. Miller (2012) suggests that the input and output processes involve exchange, while the throughput process involves feedback.

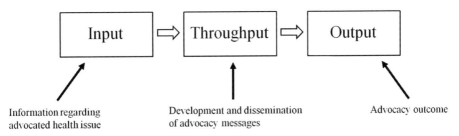

Figure 2.2: System processes shaping the Health Communication Advocacy Model.

The input and output processes in a permeable system should involve an exchange between the system and its environment. There is an exchange because the input for the system was taken from the environment and the output affects the environment. For example, a company may see a demand for paper and use trees (input) to make paper for consumers (output). In this example, the output may positively or negatively affect the environment. For instance, the former may occur when consumers get their demanded paper, but the latter may occur if trees were wastefully chopped down or if production resulted in chemical pollution. In the Health Communication Advocacy Model, however, the exchange is beneficial for the environment because the output (i.e., advocacy outcome) is intended to help the constituents of the environment, such as populations affected by the advocated health issue. To reiterate, the exchange in the Health Communication Advocacy Model would involve information regarding the advocated health issue (input) and the advocacy outcome (output). For example, the input may be statistical evidence about industrial chemical pollution and health risks (see e.g., McKenzie, Witter, Newman, & Adgate, 2012) and the output may be the implementation of industrial regulation.

The throughput process in a permeable system should involve feedback (Miller, 2012). There are two forms of feedback: corrective feedback and growth feedback. Corrective feedback, also known as negative or deviation-reducing feedback, involves monitoring for deviations from the intended goal and addressing those deviations so the system can maintain progress. For example, if the campaign team using the Health Communication Advocacy Model realized during pre-testing of messages (see Chapter 7) that audiences may not understand the advocacy message, the team may refine the message so that it would be clearer for audience to comprehend. In so doing, the team avoids deviation from the intended goal (i.e., successful advocacy campaign) and is able to maintain progression toward that goal while adhering to the model.

Growth feedback, also known as positive or deviation-amplifying feedback, involves changing a system so that the system may be improved. For example, if a campaign team utilizing the Health Communication Advocacy Model determines that advocacy messages were not adequately disseminated to youth audiences, the team may improve future advocacy efforts by paying more attention to youth audiences. In contrast to corrective feedback, growth feedback aims to improve the system for future operations, whereas corrective feedback aims to reduce deviations from current progress.

System Properties

To recap, according to systems theory, components in a system are characterized by hierarchical ordering, are interdependent, and are permeable. Because of these characteristics, a system's processes involve exchange during the input-output process and feedback during the throughput process. Based on these characteristics of system components and related processes, four properties can be inferred from open systems. The properties are: holism, equifinality, negative entropy, and requisite variety (Miller, 2012).

A holistic system is a system in which the sum of the system's parts functions better than the parts working individually. For example, in an organization, individuals may be productive working by themselves, but these individuals may be even more productive if they collaborate together and brainstorm creative ideas (Miller, 2012). Likewise, the components or phases in the Health Communication Advocacy Model may produce something beneficial individually, such as advocacy messages (from Phase 2). However, when all the components in the model work together, the output will be better; there may be potential health policy change. The model is holistic because its components are interdependent.

Equifinality means that that there are multiple ways to reach the same goal. For example, there may be various ways to get the legislature to implement health policy change. An advocate may focus more on communicating with people with relevant health issues and spend less time with the media during the advocacy campaign. Alternatively, an advocate may decide to focus more on engaging with the media and invest less time on communicating with people with relevant health issues. In any case, equifinality suggests that any of these approaches, if executed well, would lead to the same goal—a successful advocacy campaign. Equifinality also applies to the numerous possible channels/outlets that may be used in disseminating advocacy messages. For example, one may communicate advocacy messages to audiences through the radio, television news (see Wallack & Dorfman, 1996), or social media (see Valenzuela, 2013). According to the concept of equifinality, an advocacy campaign may use any or combinations of these channels/outlets and still achieve a successful advocacy campaign. Because the Health Communication Advocacy Model has the property of equifinality, campaign teams may utilize the model in a variety of ways to reach the same goal.

Entropy refers to the propensity for a closed system to deteriorate. Conversely, negative entropy refers to a system's ability to survive and be effective (Miller, 2012). The Health Communication Advocacy Model has the property of negative entropy because the model has permeable components. Thus, the model is able to adapt to situational changes and survive as a system. For instance, during pre-testing of messages, if audiences do not respond well to advocacy messages, the model allows for the advocacy team to redevelop those messages. This situational adaptability positions the model toward survival as a useful tool for advocacy teams. On the other hand, if a campaign model is closed and cannot respond to audience reactions and situational changes, the model likely will cease to be effective. For example, if audiences do not respond well to draft advocacy messages but the campaign model being used insists that the messages continue to be implemented, it is likely that audiences will not support the advocacy effort and the campaign will be unsuccessful. As another example, if a campaign model does not recommend pre-testing or evaluation of messages, ineffective messages may be disseminated and the campaign may be compromised. The Health Communication Advocacy Model avoids these pitfalls because it is open and adaptable to situational changes.

Requisite variety refers to the assumption that the processes within a system need to be as complex as the system's environment in order to effectively react to that environment (Miller, 2012). The political environment of an advocacy campaign can be quite complex; it may involve complicated health issues with challenging solutions and difficult/unreceptive audiences. Thus, an advocacy team should follow a model that has the requisite processes to manage the environment accordingly. The Health Communication Advocacy Model presents a complex process that addresses health issues with complicated solutions through formative research and strategies that are designed to persuade challenging and often unreceptive audiences to consider and adopt the advocated position.

Summary

The Health Communication Advocacy Model is grounded in systems theory, a metatheory that describes how a system works. Systems theory advances the perspective that a system needs to be open in order to grow, adapt, and survive. Although often applied to biological and organizational systems, this chapter applied systems theory to the Health Communication Advocacy Model.

The components in the Health Communication Advocacy Model adhere to hierarchical ordering, are interdependent, and are permeable. Thus, there are subsystems and supersystems in the model that are dependent on one another. These components also interact with the environment, which may include audiences and situational changes. The components in the model undergo an input-throughput-output process, during which exchange occurs in the input-output processes and feedback in the throughput process. Feedback is differentiated between corrective and growth feedback; the former monitors for deviations from the system's goal and addresses those deviations, while the latter changes a system so that future operations may improve. From these characteristics and processes of the system, four system properties are inferred including: holism, equifinality, negative entropy, and requisite variety. A holistic system is one in which the sum of its parts functions better than the parts working individually. Equifinality posits that there are multiple ways to reach a goal. Negative entropy refers to an open and adaptable system's ability to survive and be effective. Requisite variety refers to the assumption that the processes within a system need to be as complex as the system's environment in order to effectively react to that environment.

Now that the theoretical foundation of the Health Communication Advocacy Model has been expounded, we explore each phase of the model in the following chapters. Progressing through each chapter encourages a better understanding of how an effective health advocacy campaign works. The next chapter examines the beginning of the model, Phase 1, which addresses the assembling of an advocacy team.

References

Gassmann, O., Enkel, E., & Chesbrough, H. (2010). The future of open innovation. *R&D Management, 40*(3), 213–221. doi: 10.1111/j.1467-9310.2010.00605.x

Haas, E. J., & Mattson, M. (2015). *Integrating metatheory, theory, and qualitative methodology: A practical approach to enhance the research interview.* Lanham, MD: Lexington.

Mattson, M. (1999). Toward a reconceptualization of communication cues to action in the health belief model: HIV test counseling. *Communications Monographs, 66*(3), 240–265. doi: 10.1080/03637759909376476

McKenzie, L. M., Witter, R. Z., Newman, L. S., & Adgate, J. L. (2012). Human health risk assessment of air emissions from development of unconventional natural gas resources. *Science of the Total Environment, 424,* 79–87. doi: 10.1016/j.scitotenv.2012.02.018

Miller, K. (2012). *Organizational communication: Approaches and processes* (6th ed.). Boston, MA: Wadsworth, Cengage Learning.

Valenzuela, S. (2013). Unpacking the use of social media for protest behavior: The roles of information, opinion expression, and activism. *American Behavioral Scientist, 57*(7), 920–942. doi: 10.1177/0002764213479375

Von Bertalanffy, L. (1968). *General system theory: Foundations, development, applications.* New York: George Braziller.

Wallack, L., & Dorfman, L. (1996). Media advocacy: A strategy for advancing policy and promoting health. *Health Education & Behavior*, 23(3), 293–317. doi: 10.1177/109019819602300303

Zhao, S. (1991). Metatheory, metamethod, meta-data-analysis: What, why, and how? *Sociological perspectives*, 34(3), 377–390. doi: 10.2307/1389517

· 3 ·

ASSEMBLING THE TEAM

Before a health advocacy initiative can begin, an advocacy team must first be assembled. The members in an advocacy team may include health issue experts, community partners, public health and/or communication specialists, and a lobbyist. Each of these members plays a significant and unique role in advancing an advocacy team toward its goal.

Health Issue Experts

Health issue experts are professionals with specialized knowledge in a particular health area. For instance, an expert about ovarian cancer would be a gynecologic oncologist (see e.g., Earle et al., 2006). Other examples of experts include physiotherapists for amputee rehabilitation, nurses for palliative care, surgeons for surgical procedures, and so on. Patients also can be health issue experts because of their knowledge of and experience with the health issue. The benefits they can bring to the team are primarily twofold: health experts can lend credibility to the team and can help to avoid making medical-related mistakes.

Health issue experts can transfer their credibility to a group. This is well supported by halo-effect studies reported in psychology and marketing literature (see e.g., Leuthesser, Kohli, & Harich, 1995). The reputation of health experts such as doctors can build the reputation of a group. When reputation is strong and the message source is believable, the recipient of the message is more likely to have a favorable initial hearing and is more likely to be influenced by the message (Herbig & Milewicz, 1995). Furthermore, should recipients be unmotivated to process messages, the presence of experts serves as a favorable cue for their evaluation of the messages (Petty & Cacioppo, 1984). Thus, health experts help boost the credibility of an assembled team.

Experts can also help the group to avoid medical-related mistakes. Because of their expertise, medical experts are able to detect or anticipate detrimental mistakes that might occur during the course of health advocacy planning. For instance, health advocacy planners might want to embark upon a campaign about organ donation but might know very little about the risks and complications involved in the organ donation process (e.g., Ommen, Winston, & Murphy, 2006; cf. Hartmann, Fauchald, Westlie, Brekke, & Holdaas, 2003), thus health issue experts should be recruited to advise advocacy planners against making potentially detrimental medical assumptions. The use of experts is increasingly important in contributing to policy and decision-making (see e.g., Fick et al., 2003; Pauwelyn, 2002).

Community Partners

Pivotal to the success of advocacy movements is collaboration. Collaboration can be achieved through engaging with community partners, which may include unions, clubs, associations, health departments, clinics, universities, and so on (see e.g., Krieger et al., 2002). By enlisting the help of community partners, advocacy efforts can benefit from pooled resources, diversity, wider range of skilled personnel, and farther reach in campaigns. When community partners cooperate to work towards a mutual goal, they can become a larger unit known as a coalition, which is an assembly of individuals from various organizations who work together towards a shared goal (Sabatier, 1988; see also Weible et al., 2011). An advocacy team may choose to embark on setting up their own coalition (see Mizrahi, 2001, for a discussion on such a task), or the team can opt to work with pre-existing coalitions instead. There are many benefits of working with a coalition, including acquiring of resources, integrating new ideas, perspectives, and technologies, and having a broader understanding of problems (Roberts-DeGennaro, 1987).

The effectiveness of coalitions in bringing about changes in health issues is supported by research. For example, in Louisiana, the community-based coalition—"Shots for Tots"—mobilized people from healthcare agencies and community organizations to work towards the goal of having 90% of all 2-year-olds immunized within the Lafayette region. Representatives from healthcare included nurses, a public healthcare clinic, and the Office of Public Health, while those from community organizations included the Junior League, Medical Auxiliary, Kiwanis Club, and Rotary International. Healthcare representatives such as nurses were engaged in administering immunizations and were actively promoting the importance of timely immunization to the parents of toddlers. Through federal funding, "Shots for Tots" clinics were able to provide markedly-lower vaccination fees. Community organizations played a role by providing funds and service hours for media campaigns that promoted the plans of the coalition, such as the use of public service announcements, banners, billboards, and various advertising strategies. Their collaboration was successful, and the Lafayette region experienced an increase in immunization rates for 2-year-olds (Broussard & Blankenship, 1996).

The effectiveness of coalitions spans across many different kinds of health issues. For instance, the Bootheel Heart Health Project in southeastern Missouri reported an increase in cholesterol screening and a decrease in physical inactivity in areas that had participating coalitions (Brownson, 1996). Other health concerns that coalitions have helped address include smoking, alcohol consumption, student physical activity, and healthcare service access (Roussos & Fawcett, 2000).

Because of the effectiveness of coalitions, it is encouraged that advocacy movements work in concert with coalitions. As the previous examples illustrate, coalitions can promote awareness of efforts that positively influence health issues and can be instrumental in instilling change towards healthful behaviors.

Public Health/Communication Specialists

According to the American Public Health Association (2007), specialists in public health focus on three issues: the prevention of disease and illness among groups of people, the formulation of public policy regarding health concerns, and community health surveillance, which involves monitoring diseases and researching causes and cures for diseases and other health matters. With this understanding, it is clear that public health specialists are vital members in the advocacy process, as they are trained in dealing with community health and the public policy governing community health. One method public health specialists use is social marketing, which is defined as the use of commercial marketing principles to address social issues (Kotler & Lee, 2008). However, because public health specialists have an incomplete understanding of social marketing (Grier & Bryant, 2005), public health professionals might find it challenging to reach out to target populations. Furthermore, the concept of social marketing itself has come under scrutiny. One criticism is that campaigns using social marketing have been unsuccessful in producing or maintaining desired behavioral changes (MacStravic, 2000). Other scholars have added that social marketing does not adequately consider the message design process, and messages are not tailored sufficiently to meet audience needs (Mattson & Basu, 2010a, 2010b; Mattson & Hall, 2011). Thus, it is imperative that communication specialists join forces with public health specialists in campaign design, implementation, and evaluation.

Lobbyists

Lobbyists are professionals who attempt to persuade legislators into policy change. Lobbyists often are affiliated with businesses, and in 2008 a total of $3.97 billion was spent on lobbying (Vidal, Draca, & Fons-Rosen, 2012). Fundamentally, the lobbyist acts as a mediator between a person or group (i.e., the client) calling for change in policy via the legislator. Because the client's interest most likely will not be in tandem with the legislator, the lobbyist is hired to intercede. The client proposes its interest to the lobbyist, who then attempts to persuade the legislator, who then may or may not agree to act on policy change. The need for a lobbyist from the perspective of a client may be quite substantial: the lobbyist has a reputation and connection with the policy community that the client does not have, and the client usually has a paucity of policy activity, political knowledge, and information on how the government makes decisions (Kersh, 2000).

In an attempt to define the term "lobbyist," Thomas and Hrebenar (2009) suggested that the term describes:

A person designated by an interest group to facilitate influencing public policy in that group's favor by performing one or more of the following for the group: (1) directly contacting public officials; (2) monitoring political and governmental activity; (3) advising on political strategies and tactics; and (4) developing and orchestrating the group's lobbying effort. (pp. 135)

Let's further expound on these lobbyist actions. In contacting politicians, a lobbyist seeks to build rapport with policymakers by gaining access to them. To monitor activity, a lobbyist observes politicians and acquires information about them. For instance, what is the politician's background? What is the politician's position on certain issues? The observations can be as subtle as what sitting posture the politician adopts when disinterested in a topic. Monitoring is a form of political intelligence, a gathering of information on what strategies would work best in a lobbyist's and/or a client's favor. It also is about keeping up to date with laws and regulations that may be of concern. In regards to the advising function of a lobbyist, it is crucial to understand that the lobbyist is not an advocate, but an advisor to the advocate, namely, the client. A lobbyist provides a client access to legislators and advises how the client should go about persuading the legislators. Additionally, the lobbyist can encourage strategies such as the formation of grassroots groups to urge legislators into taking action. A lobbyist also can advise on coalition building, which is the rallying of many different organizations to stand united for one common interest (McGrath, 2005).

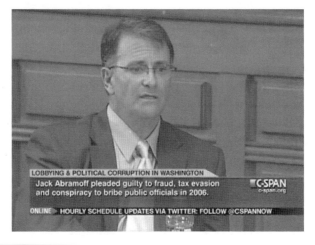

Video Library 1: Jack Abramoff case (C-Span, 2011)

Increasingly lobbying is met with negative reception. There is mistrust and disdain by journalists and the public towards lobbying, due in part to the exposed malpractices of lobbyists and the perceived associated corruption in lobbying (Hamer & El Nahas, 2006; McGrath, 2005). For example, a Republican lobbyist named Jack Abramoff pled guilty to charges of tax evasion, fraud, and corruption on January 3, 2006. He was involved in bribing officials, giving free meals to politicians at his restaurant, and he allegedly took payments from clients without following up with action. These, and many more malpractices, resulted in an order for him to pay $22 million in restitution and serve 70 months in prison.

Although such instances of offenses and apparent negative attitudes toward lobbyists exist, the positive contribution that legitimate and proper lobbying provides should not be overlooked. Furthermore, lobbying is a common practice in the political system, much of which is conducted properly (McGrath, 2007). Thus, our interest is not in the debate or furor over scandals and conspiracies, but in the proper function of legitimate lobbying. As a final consideration, there are certain preferences for what this lobbying role should be called, ranging from "lobbyist" to "government affairs" to "public affairs." This range of terms stems from the negative connotations associated with "lobbyist," and also is due to the arguments over what the role encompasses (McGrath, 2005). However, since the term "lobbyist" is increasingly accepted, and because it is widely associated with Washington instead of European politics (McGrath, 2005), this book uses the terms lobbyist and lobbying, referring to the person and activity, respectively, that mediate between client and legislator to promote policy change.

Craft Position Statement

When an advocacy team has been assembled, the team should decide when to meet periodically to discuss the advocacy progress. Responsibilities also should be assigned to each member according to their skills. If the advocacy team decides fundraising is necessary for the advocacy effort, the team will have to discuss fundraising strategies. It also is essential for the advocacy team to formulate a position statement on the health issue. The position statement contains both the stance of the team regarding the health concern and the goal the team is reaching for. For example, the advocacy team Professor Mattson was involved with decided that their position statement would be that amputees should receive parity in health insurance coverage for prosthetics. This position statement contained their shared belief about what insurance benefits amputees should expect, and the team used this statement as their goal to work towards. Often an advocacy team's position statement involves a legislative bill or proposed law, as was the case for Professor Mattson's advocacy team, which got the bill, HB1140, to pass into law (Mattson, 2010). However, advocacy teams need not restrict themselves to just one position statement; they can have multiple statements as long as there are no contradictions or conflicting positions, and if multiple statements could be advanced just as effectively and resourcefully as a single statement. For instance, in response to the health issue of childhood obesity (see e.g., Ebbeling, Pawlak, & Ludwig, 2002; Swinburn et al., 2011) an advocacy team might desire to champion the promotion of healthy foods in schools, the restriction of direct food marketing to children, and the implementation of dietary education. However, having so many positional statements might be too daunting and challenging for the team to handle, and the team might fare better by adopting one position statement, such as dietary education. Positional statements are very important in advocacy movements, and it is imperative that a team decides what their position statement or statements will be before they proceed forward with their advocacy campaign.

Summary

When convening an advocacy team, the following are crucial members who would contribute to the advocacy effort: (1) health issue experts—for their knowledge, expertise, and advice about the most appropriate and beneficial approach to tackle the health issue; (2) community partners—for the access they can provide for campaigns to reach local communities and relevant audiences (3) public health/communication specialists—who will be instrumental in planning, designing, and implementing the advocacy campaign; and possibly a (4) lobbyist—who, if necessary, helps engage networks and provides meeting and negotiation opportunities with politicians and legislators.

Once the team is assembled, the team would need to decide when to meet periodically to discuss advocacy progress and assign responsibilities to team members. If fundraising is necessary for the advocacy effort, the team would have to discuss fundraising strategies. The advocacy team also would need to craft a positional statement, which is the stance they take concerning a health issue. This statement also serves as the goal for the advocacy team to achieve. When the team determines its positional statement, the team can commence with Phase 2 of the Health Communication Advocacy Model.

References

American Public Health Association (2007). *What is public health? Our commitment to safe, healthy communities.* Washington, DC: Author.

Broussard, L. A., & Blankenship, F. B. (1996). Shots for tots: Louisiana's infant immunization initiative. *Journal for Specialists in Pediatric Nursing, 1*(3), 113–116. doi: 10.1111/j.1744-6155.1996.tb00013.x

Brownson, R. C. (1996). Preventing cardiovascular disease through community-based risk reduction: The Bootheel Heart Health Project. *American Journal of Public Health, 86*(2), 206–213. Retrieved from http://www.ajph.org/

C-SPAN. (2011). Jack Abramoff on political corruption. Available from www.c-span.org/

Earle, C. C., Schrag, D., Neville, B. A., Yabroff, K. R., Topor, M., Fahey, A., ... & Warren, J. L. (2006). Effect of surgeon specialty on processes of care and outcomes for ovarian cancer patients. *Journal of the National Cancer Institute, 98*(3), 172–180. doi: 10.1093/jnci/djj019

Ebbeling, C. B., Pawlak, D. B., & Ludwig, D. S. (2002). Childhood obesity: Public-health crisis, common sense cure. *The Lancet, 360*(9331), 473–482. doi: 10.1016/S0140-6736(02)09678-2

Fick, D. M., Cooper, J. W., Wade, W. E., Waller, J. L., Maclean, J. R., & Beers, M. H. (2003). Updating the Beers criteria for potentially inappropriate medication use in older adults: Results of a US consensus panel of experts. *Archives of Internal Medicine, 163*(22), 2716–2724. doi: 10.1001/archinte.163.22.2716

Grier, S., & Bryant, C. A. (2005). Social marketing in public health. *Annual Review of Public Health, 26*(1), 319–339. doi:10.1146/annurev.publhealth.26.021304.144610

Hamer, R. A., & El Nahas, A. M. (2006). The burden of chronic kidney disease: is rising rapidly worldwide. *BMJ: British Medical Journal, 332*(7541), 563. Retrieved from http://group.bmj.com/

Hartmann, A., Fauchald, P., Westlie, L., Brekke, I. B., & Holdaas, H. (2003). The risk of living kidney donation. *Nephrology Dialysis Transplantation, 18*(5), 871–873. doi: 10.1093/ndt/gfg069

Herbig, P., & Milewicz, J. (1995). The relationship of reputation and credibility to brand success. *Journal of Consumer Marketing, 12*(4), 5–10. doi: 10.1108/07363769510795697

Kersh, R. (2000). State autonomy & civil society: The lobbyist connection. *Critical Review, 14*(2–3), 237–258. doi: 10.1080/08913810008443559

Kotler, P., & Lee, N. R. (2008). *Social marketing: Influencing behaviors for good* (3rd ed.). Thousand Oaks, CA: Sage.

Krieger, J., Allen, C., Cheadle, A., Ciske, S., Schier, J. K., Senturia, K., & Sullivan, M. (2002). Using community-based participatory research to address social determinants of health:

Lessons learned from Seattle Partners for Healthy Communities. *Health Education & Behavior, 29*(3), 361–382. doi: 10.1177/109019810202900307

Leuthesser, L., Kohli, C. S., & Harich, K. R. (1995). Brand equity: The halo effect measure. *European Journal of Marketing, 29*(4), 57–66. doi: 10.1108/03090569510086657

MacStravic, S. (2000). The missing links in social marketing. *Journal of Health Communication, 5*(3), 255–263. doi: 10.1080/10810730050131424

Mattson, M. (2010). Health advocacy by accident and discipline. *Health Communication, 25*(6–7), 622–624. doi: 10.1080/10410236.2010.49684

Mattson, M., & Basu, A. (2010a). Center for disease control's diethylstilbestrol update: A case for effective operationalization of messaging in social marketing practice. *Health Promotion Practice, 11*(4), 580–588. doi: 10.1177/1524839908324785

Mattson, M., & Basu, A. (2010b). The message development tool: A case for effective operationalization of messaging in social marketing practice. *Health Marketing Quarterly, 27*(3), 275–290. doi: 10.1080/07359683.2010.495305

Mattson, M., & Hall, J. G. (2011). *Health as communication nexus*. Dubuque, IA: Kendall Hunt.

McGrath, C. (2005) *Lobbying in Washington, London, and Brussels: The persuasive communication of political issues.* Lewiston, NY: Edwin Mellen Press.

McGrath, C. (2007). Lobbying and the 2006 U.S. midterm elections. *Journal of Public Affairs, 7*(2), 192–203. doi: 10.1002/pa.257

Mizrahi, T. B. (2001). Complexities of coalition building: Leaders' successes, strategies, struggles, and solutions. *Social Work, 46*(1), 63–78. Retrieved from http://www.oxfordjournals.org/

Ommen, E. S., Winston, J. A., & Murphy, B. (2006). Medical risks in living kidney donors: Absence of proof is not proof of absence. *Clinical Journal of the American Society of Nephrology, 1*(4), 885–895. doi: 10.2215/CJN.00840306

Pauwelyn, J. (2002). The use of experts in WTO dispute settlement. *International and Comparative Law Quarterly, 51*(02), 325–364. Retrieved from http://www.jstor.org/stable/3663232

Petty, R. E., & Cacioppo, J. T. (1984). Source factors and the elaboration likelihood model of persuasion. *Advances in Consumer Research, 11*(1), 668–672. Retrieved from http://www.acrweb.org/

Roberts-DeGennaro, M. (1987). Patterns of exchange relationships in building a coalition. *Administration in Social Work, 11*(1), 59–67. doi: 10.1300/J147v11n01_06

Roussos, S., & Fawcett, S. B. (2000). A review of collaborative partnerships as a strategy for improving community health. *Annual Review of Public Health, 21*(1), 369–402. Retrieved from http://arjournals.annualreviews.org

Sabatier, P. A. (1988). An advocacy coalition framework of policy change and the role of policy-oriented learning therein. *Policy Sciences, 21*(2–3), 12–168. Retrieved from http://www.jstor.org/stable/4532139

Swinburn, B. A., Sacks, G., Hall, K. D., McPherson, K., Finegood, D. T., Moodie, M. L., & Gortmaker, S. L. (2011). The global obesity pandemic: Shaped by global drivers and local environments. *The Lancet, 378*(9793), 804–814. doi: 10.1016/S0140–6736(11)60813–1

Thomas, C. S., & Hrebenar, R. J. (2009). Comparing lobbying across liberal democracies: Problems, approaches and initial findings. *Journal of Comparative Politics, 2*(1), 131–142. Retrieved from http://www.jofcp.org/jcp/

Vidal, J. B. I., Draca, M., & Fons-Rosen, C. (2012). Revolving door lobbyists. *The American Economic Review, 102*(7), 3731–3748. doi: 10.1257/aer.102.7.3731

Weible, C. M., Sabatier, P. A., Jenkins-Smith, H. C., Nohrstedt, D., Henry, A., & deLeon, P. (2011). A quarter century of the advocacy coalition framework: An introduction to the special issue. *Policy Studies Journal, 39*(3), 349–360. doi:10.1111/j.1541–0072.2011.00412.x

· 4 ·

NEEDS ASSESSMENT

Before diving into an advocacy campaign, an advocacy team must first assess if an advocacy campaign is possible and warranted. An advocacy team should begin a campaign only if an advocacy effort is necessary to address a health issue and if it is possible to conduct an advocacy campaign. There may be situations when an advocacy effort is not necessary to address a health issue, such as curbing obesity because personal commitment to exercise may be more effective than a policy change that tackles obesity indirectly. Also, there may be circumstances when it is not possible to conduct an advocacy campaign, such as when there are many weaknesses in an advocacy team and many threats that deter the team from launching a campaign. To determine if an advocacy campaign is necessary and possible, an advocacy team can conduct a needs assessment. There are three parts to a comprehensive needs assessment: SWOT analysis, community asset mapping, and key informant interviews. An advocacy team can have greater confidence that an advocacy campaign is necessary and possible after the team completes these three aspects of a needs assessment.

SWOT Analysis

A SWOT analysis is a marketing tool that examines the internal and external attributes that can affect a campaign (Mattson & Hall, 2011). This analysis helps a campaign team know what the strengths and weaknesses are in a team and what environmental factors may help or challenge the team and its efforts. Ultimately, it helps a campaign team know if it is possible to conduct an advocacy campaign. SWOT is an acronym that stands for:

Strengths
Weaknesses
Opportunities
Threats

Strengths, weaknesses, opportunities, and threats are four categories that make up the SWOT analysis. Table 4.1 illustrates a SWOT analysis. Typically, a health advocacy team will fill in the SWOT analysis table with relevant items according to the categories, and the item descriptions should be brief. The upper half of the SWOT analysis table represents the internal attributes that can affect a health advocacy team and its potential campaign, and the lower half represents the external attributes that can affect a health advocacy campaign. Internal attributes are derived from within the team (e.g., experience, finances), whereas external attributes are derived from environmental factors (e.g., community support). The internal and external attributes are discussed accordingly.

Table 4.1: SWOT Analysis table.

	Helpful to achieving objective	Harmful to achieving objective
Internal Attributes (advocacy team)	Strengths **S**	Weaknesses **W**
External Attributes (environment)	Opportunities **O**	Threats **T**

Strengths and Weaknesses

Internal attributes are characteristics of an advocacy team that can affect an advocacy campaign. The strengths and weaknesses categories in the SWOT analysis are for assessing what characteristics of the advocacy team help or hinder an advocacy campaign respectively. For example, a strength of an advocacy team may be the experience of many of its members, while a weakness may be the team's limited budget. There are numerous possible strengths, including advocacy experience, abundant resources, knowledge about the health issue, expertise in graphic design and communication, experience in politics, and so on. There also are numerous possible weaknesses. Table 4.2 provides an illustration of the possible strengths and weaknesses of an advocacy team.

An advocacy team should aim to maximize strengths and minimize weaknesses. To do so, an advocacy team needs to first assess what the team is lacking in an area and/or why a particular weakness exists. For example, if a team's weakness is lack of experience in politics, the advocacy team should ask itself why this is so for the team. Is it because the team has not recruited a lobbyist? Or is it because the team's lobbyist has had very little experience with legislation? If it is the former, the advocacy team can turn the weakness into a strength by hiring a lobbyist. If it is the latter, an advocacy team may want to consider hiring a different lobbyist. Sometimes weaknesses may be interrelated. For instance, a weakness such as lack of experience in politics may exist because the advocacy team has not recruited a lobbyist, and the reason for not recruiting a lobbyist may be because the team has insufficient funds to hire a lobbyist. In such situations, a team may resolve one weakness if it first addresses the root weakness.

Sometimes, an advocacy team cannot abolish all weaknesses. For example, an advocacy team may not be able to recruit anyone who is proficient in graphic design, and the lack of such a member may be a lingering weakness. In such a situation, an advocacy team must make do with the weakness and approach advocacy in a way that does not require graphic design. So instead of using printed banners that involve a more complicated graphic design, an advocacy team may make do with simple, hand-painted banners for a rally. Or, instead of using computer animation for a video promotion of the advocated health issue, an advocacy team may use real actors and actresses for the video, such as in testimonial videos. An advocacy team also should focus on and emphasize the strengths that the team has in order to compensate for the weaknesses during the campaign.

Table 4.2: Possible strengths and weaknesses of an advocacy team.

Possible strengths and weaknesses of an advocacy team	
Strengths	Weaknesses
• Vast experience in advocacy • Research skills • Financial resources • Graphic design skills • Cohesion and teamwork • All members understand and work toward advocacy goal • Members have excellent reputation • Members who ask questions, provide feedback, and cooperate	• Lack of experience in advocacy • Limited budget • No graphic design skills • Divisiveness within team • Different perspectives on advocacy goal • Disagreements and conflicts regarding advocacy approach • Members who do not contribute • Lack of knowledge about advocated health issue

On other occasions, the SWOT analysis may reveal that there are more weaknesses than strengths. In such situations an advocacy team might want to consider withdrawing from an advocacy effort because continuing with the advocacy campaign may not be workable or worthwhile. Table 4.3 provides an illustration.

Table 4.3: More weaknesses than strengths illustration.

	Helpful to achieving objective	Harmful to achieving objective
Internal Attributes (advocacy team)	Strengths: - Members have experience in advocacy	Weaknesses: - Different ideas on what advocacy goal should be - Limited budget - Lack of knowledge on health issue
External Attributes (environment)	Opportunities	Threats

In the example illustrated in Table 4.3, the advocacy team has three weaknesses in contrast to the one strength. The weaknesses are: different ideas about what the advocacy goal should be, a limited budget, and a lack of knowledge on the advocated health issue. An advocacy campaign can be in a fragile and compromising position if members of the advocacy team have differing opinions about what the advocacy goal should be. This is because advocacy requires a concerted effort and an advocacy campaign may risk becoming unorganized and ineffective if members of an advocacy team do not agree on what the advocacy goal should be. For instance, the advocacy goal for some members of an advocacy team may be to persuade the legislature to implement policies to control food marketing targeting children (see Ebbeling, Pawlak, & Ludwig, 2002; Swinburn et al., 2011), while other members of the team may instead want the abolishment of food marketing targeting children to be the advocacy goal. In such situations, the advocacy team likely would carry out the advocacy campaign ineffectively. For instance, the advocacy team may have differing and competing messages in a rally, or some members of the team may appear unconvinced about advocacy messages crafted by other members in the team. Audiences of the rally likely will be confused by the contrasting messages. Also, audiences may not have confidence supporting an advocacy team that has members appearing unconvinced about their own team's messages.

Another weakness listed in Table 4.3 is limited budget. Having insufficient financial resources for an advocacy campaign can be detrimental to carrying out the campaign effectively. For example, the advocacy team may not be able to hire a lobbyist, who can be essential for navigating the complexities of politics. A lack of funds also can impede an advocacy campaign because it may limit, for example, the number of times an advocacy team can travel to promote awareness or the number of times a rally can be conducted. The final weakness listed on the SWOT analysis in Table 4.3 is that the team may lack knowledge about the advocated health issue. An advocacy team that does not have a comprehensive or expert knowledge about the advocated health issue may not appear credible to audiences. For instance, if an advocacy team promoting equal coverage for prosthetics across insurance plans does not have a member who is an amputee or prosthetic expert, the team may appear unconvincing if it claims that it understands what challenges amputees face in coping without prosthetic limbs.

The team members' experience in advocacy was listed as a strength in the SWOT analysis in Table 4.3. Experience in advocacy can be useful because it can enhance the credibility of the advocacy team and the experienced members may advocate more efficiently. However, there are too many weaknesses and that may overshadow the strength of the advocacy team. For example, although the team members have experience in advocacy, the members have divided opinions about what the advocacy goal should be and therefore the team's experience may not result in an effective advocacy campaign. Even if the advocacy team decides to ignore the divided opinions, the limited budget can restrict a team from carrying out advocacy effectively. Furthermore, although the team has experience in advocacy, they may not have sufficient knowledge about the current health issue to advocate effectively. Therefore, although the SWOT analysis in Table 4.3 listed one strength, the number of weaknesses eclipsed that single strength. In such a situation, it may be better for the advocacy team to withdraw and not proceed with an advocacy campaign because the campaign likely would not be carried out successfully. An advocacy team should wait for a more opportune time and conduct the SWOT analysis again to determine if the team has more strengths and fewer weaknesses at that time. When an advocacy team has much more strengths than weaknesses listed in the SWOT analysis, the team will be in a better position to proceed with an advocacy campaign. However, that also assumes that there are more opportunities than threats in the SWOT analysis. Opportunities and threats are external attributes which will be considered later.

Sometimes, having a greater quantity of strengths in the SWOT analysis may not mean that an advocacy team is in a better position to proceed with an advocacy campaign. In some cases, quality or extent of a strength or weakness can affect the decision to proceed with a campaign. Table 4.4 below provides an example of such a case.

In the SWOT analysis in Table 4.4, there is only one weakness in contrast to three strengths. However, the extent of the weakness may be so great that it may dwarf the strengths of the team. The disagreements over advocacy approaches may affect the strengths indirectly. For instance, although members of the advocacy team have skills in graphic design, the members may disagree about the look of graphic designs for the advocacy campaign. Also, experts may argue over how the health issue should be discussed or portrayed in advocacy messages. Lastly, even though there may be sufficient financial resources, the advocacy team may be so fragmented that the team cannot proceed with an advocacy campaign. In such an instance, the internal conflicts resulting from disagreements over advocacy approaches may be so damaging that the strengths of the team may be rendered null and void. Therefore, there are times when the quality or extent of a strength or weakness can be significant enough to determine whether it is possible to conduct an advocacy campaign.

Table 4.4: Example of a problematic weakness.

		Helpful to achieving objective	**Harmful** to achieving objective
Internal Attributes (advocacy team)		Strengths: - Members with skills in graphic design - Financial resources - Members who are experts in the health issue	Weaknesses: - Disagreements over advocacy approaches
External Attributes (environment)		Opportunities *O*	Threats *T*

Opportunities and Threats

External attributes are environmental factors that can affect an advocacy campaign. The opportunities and threats categories in the SWOT analysis are for assessing what environmental factors advance or impede an advocacy campaign, respectively. For example, an opportunity may be having community support, or having a network through coalitions. A coalition is an alliance of people from various organizations who work together toward a shared goal (Sabatier, 1988; see also Weible et al., 2011). The extensive network of a coalition can help an advocacy team reach out to relevant audiences efficiently. Examples of threats are competing campaigns or messages, resistant audiences, and an impending deadline. Deadlines are important as an advocacy effort may not be effective after the deadline. For example, if an advocacy team has a deadline that is before the commencement of the legislative session or budget cycle, but fails to meet the deadline, the team's efforts may be compromised because legislators would be preoccupied and unable to attend to the team during that busy period (see Gregrich, 2003). An advocacy team that has little time remaining before the deadline is unlikely to have time for important tasks, such as conducting formative research on the advocated health issue and on target audiences, planning and developing advocacy messages, disseminating advocacy messages strategically, and correcting messages when some of the messages are not successful. Therefore, if an advocacy team attempts to advocate despite having insufficient time, the advocacy effort likely would be a perfunctory and ineffective one. Future advocacy efforts also may become more difficult because advocacy audiences may be hesitant to support an advocacy effort that previously was unimpressive. Table 4.5 below provides a list of possible opportunities and threats for an advocacy team.

Table 4.5: Possible opportunities and threats for an advocacy team.

Possible opportunities and threats for an advocacy team	
Opportunities	Threats
• Community support • Networks • Media support • Receptive audiences • Adequate time • No competing campaigns or messages • Permission from shopping malls to set up a petition booth inside the mall • Other organizations promoting awareness about the advocated health issue as well (e.g., cancer coalitions)	• Lack of support from community • Lack of network • Audiences do not have much prior knowledge about the advocated health issue • Impending deadline • Resistant audiences • Competing campaigns that advocate for other issues, such as better employment policies, tax reductions, etc. • Competing advocacy campaigns that are health-related (e.g., cancer-treatment affordability)

Similar to the illustrations for strengths and weaknesses, an advocacy team is more likely able to proceed with an advocacy campaign if the number of opportunities is greater than the number of threats. However, unlike strengths and weaknesses, sometimes there is little that an advocacy team can do to maximize opportunities and minimize threats. For example, it is beyond an advocacy team's control that advocacy audiences have little prior knowledge about the advocated health issue. But often it is possible for an advocacy team to maximize or minimize opportunities or threats. For example, an advocacy team may actively seek out collaborations and networks by calling or emailing relevant organizations. An advocacy team also may relocate to avoid competing campaigns.

When all categories of the SWOT analysis have been assessed, an advocacy team determines whether the team is in a good position to proceed with an advocacy campaign or to withdraw. An advocacy team should continue with an advocacy effort only if there are more helpful attributes than there are harmful ones, or if some helpful attributes are so advantageous that the harmful attributes become relatively benign. Table 4.6 below is an illustration of a completed SWOT analysis table that shows an advocacy campaign is likely feasible.

Table 4.6: Example of a completed SWOT analysis table.

	Helpful to achieving objective	Harmful to achieving objective
Internal Attributes (advocacy team)	Strengths: - Financial resources - Members who are experts in health issue - Experience in advocacy	Weaknesses: - Lacking members with skills in graphic design
External Attributes (environment)	Opportunities: - Networks - Adequate time - No competing campaign that is health-related or similar	Threats: - Audiences do not have prior knowledge about the advocated health issue

The depicted scenario in Table 4.6 suggests that an advocacy campaign is feasible. There are many more helpful attributes than there are harmful ones, and a few of the helpful attributes are crucial for an advocacy campaign. For instance, there is adequate time for an advocacy campaign, which is very important because an advocacy campaign requires sufficient time to be well executed. Also, there is no competing campaign that is health-related or similar, which means that the advocacy team will have an easier task of reaching out to its audiences, particularly legislators, as the legislators will not be inundated with many campaign requests.

In addition to having more helpful attributes, the harmful attributes are not very threatening and easily can be overcome. For instance, although the weakness of the advocacy team is that it lacks members with skills in graphic design, this weakness is not debilitating. The advocacy team could circumvent the weakness by avoiding communication mediums that require graphic designs, such as computer-animated videos or elaborately-designed posters or banners. The advocacy team could use alternative approaches, such as a video with real actors or actresses, or a banner designed by hand. Because the advocacy team has financial resources, the weakness also can be overcome by hiring individuals who are proficient in graphic design. Another harmful attribute was the threat that audiences do not have prior knowledge about the advocated health issue. This problem also is not detrimental and can be overcome. If audiences do not have prior knowledge about the health issue, an advocacy team can address this lack of knowledge by explaining the health issue in its advocacy messages to audiences. However, an advocacy team should explain the health issue in a brief and succinct manner because it is important to maintain the interest of audiences and not bore audiences with too many details (Chapter 6 discusses strategies in developing advocacy messages that will capture the attention of audiences). In some cases, the situation in which audiences do not have prior knowledge on the advocated health issue may be more of an opportunity than a threat. First, the audiences may not have any preconceived biases against a particular health issue and may be more open to hearing about it. Second, the audiences may be more curious and interested to know how they may be susceptible to the health issue or how the health issue may affect them. Thus, this threat and the previously listed weakness do not pose significant danger to an advocacy campaign and can be easily overcome. Given these considerations, an advocacy team with such a SWOT analysis can be confident that the team may be in a good position to proceed with an advocacy campaign.

The SWOT analysis is useful for an advocacy team to determine what internal and external attributes can be helpful or harmful for an advocacy campaign. Internal attributes are the strengths and weaknesses of an advocacy team that can affect an advocacy campaign. External attributes are environmental opportunities and threats that can affect an advocacy campaign. Attributes that are helpful include strengths of an advocacy team and environmental opportunities. Attributes that are harmful include weaknesses of an advocacy team and environmental threats. An advocacy team should maximize helpful attributes and minimize harmful attributes in order to increase the feasibility of an advocacy campaign. If there are more significant helpful attributes than there are harmful attributes, an advocacy team may be more confident that an advocacy campaign is feasible. If an advocacy team ascertains that an advocacy campaign is feasible, the SWOT analysis also would have helped the advocacy team to identify and take advantage of its strengths and opportunities during the campaign. If an advocacy team determines that an advocacy campaign is not feasible because of the results of the SWOT analysis, the advocacy team is able to avoid a costly and ineffective campaign. After an advocacy team conducts a SWOT analysis and ascertains that an advocacy campaign is feasible, the team still needs to conduct community asset mapping and key informant interviews to determine if the team should proceed with an advocacy campaign.

Community Asset Mapping

An advocacy team should know what resources are available in a community because the team can make use of the available resources. For instance, if there is a coalition within a community that has a large network, an advocacy team may take advantage of the network by collaborating with the coalition. An advocacy team also should know what resources are lacking in a community because the team may want to address the lack of resources as a supporting argument in advocacy messages. For example, if an advocacy team is advocating for the allocation of more state resources for building cancer-treatment facilities, the advocacy team may enhance its position by emphasizing in advocacy messages that the state has very few cancer-treatment facilities. In order to know what resources are available or lacking in a community, an advocacy team can use the community asset mapping technique. Community asset mapping is a technique that involves mapping out the resources within a community (Griffin & Farris, 2010), and can be useful for the purposes of advocacy (Healthy City, 2012). For instance, an advocacy team may map out where the exercise facilities are in a university campus if it is advocating for more exercise facilities to be built in schools. There are four ways to do community asset mapping: focus groups, interviews, surveys, or community walks (Healthy City, 2012).

Focus Groups

A focus group is a small gathering of homogeneous people assembled by an individual who is seeking more information for a specific inquiry (see Guest, Namey, & Mitchell, 2013). Chapter 7 discusses focus groups at greater length. Within the context of community asset mapping, it will suffice to know that a focus group involves assembling community members to discuss the resources in their community. An advocacy team may recruit about eight to twelve participants for a focus group session, and the participants should be representative of the community. For instance, if a community is mostly comprised of African Americans and Hispanics, then focus groups should be representative of African American and Hispanic participants. An advocacy team should provide focus group participants with a large map that charts out a simple but accurate layout of the community. An advocacy team should inform participants what resources the team is looking for so that the participants may mark out the locations of those resources. An advocacy team may provide colorful stickers or pens for participants to mark out locations according to a color scheme, which is the use of colors to represent different items. For instance, an advocacy team may write a legend on the side of the community map that indicates the color blue for churches, yellow for schools, green for shopping places. An advocacy team may use such a color scheme to find out where many people convene so that the team may advocate in those locations. Figure 4.1 illustrates an example of community asset mapping:

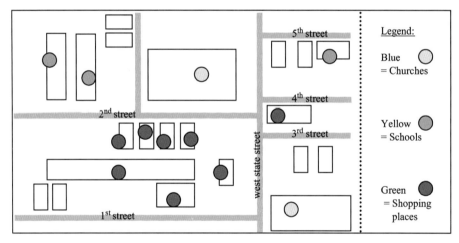

Figure 4.1: Example of community asset mapping using colorful stickers.

In the example illustrated in Figure 4.1, most people seem to convene around 2nd street and therefore an advocacy group may want to advocate in that area. An advocacy team may decide to advocate inside a building such as a shopping mall, but doing so requires permission from the building management and gaining that approval can be challenging. Alternatively, the advocacy team may advocate in an open public space which is near a populated area. Accordingly, the advocacy team should gauge where the most strategic location to advocate is based on the relative proximity of other convening points.

That is to say, the strategic location on the map should be near as many colored stickers as possible.

Figure 4.2 shows two possible strategic locations for advocacy. Point A may be an advantageous location because it is situated near two schools and is across the street from a church and several shopping places. Therefore, Point A may be a good strategic location because the advocacy team may be able to reach out to three different types of audiences. Point B also may be advantageous because it is near many shopping places and is across the street from a church and another shopping area. Point B also is near the intersections of several roadways, and thus there likely is good visibility for the advocacy campaign as there will be many vehicles driving by. For instance, if the advocacy team conducts a rally at Point B, vehicle drivers that pass by may become intrigued by the signboards, banners, and noise of the rally and decide to take a look at what is happening. However, unlike Point A, Point B may not be as effective in reaching out to schools because it is situated some distance away from schools. Therefore, the advocacy team may risk losing a substantial number of student audiences if it decides to advocate at Point B. However, if students are not a target audience for the advocacy team, Point B's distance from schools should not pose a problem. Instead, the distance away from schools may serve as an advantage in such a situation because it helps filter out people who are not relevant audiences for the advocacy campaign. Therefore, an advocacy team should take into account proximity, visibility, and target audiences in assessing the best location to advocate in a community.

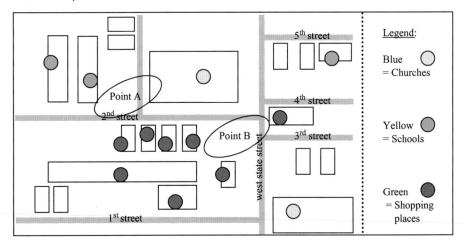

Figure 4.2: Example of possible strategic locations.

Interviews

Another approach to community asset mapping is conducting interviews (Healthy City, 2012). An interview involves asking a person questions in order to gain understanding on a particular subject (see Lindlof & Taylor, 2011). An advocacy team representative may interview members of a community to find out where certain resources are located within the community. Similar to focus groups, the participants recruited for interviews should be representative of the community. For instance, if there are many African Americans within the community, the interviews should be comprised mostly of African American participants. The participants also should be members of the community because they may have the best knowledge of where community assets are located. There is no fixed number of interviews that must be conducted; interviews should be conducted until saturation is reached (see Guest et al., 2013). Saturation occurs when responses from additional interviews repeat previous responses, are predictable, and do not provide new information. The interviewer should aim to build rapport quickly with participants so that the participants feel comfortable sharing their opinions (DiCicco-Bloom & Crabtree, 2006; Healthy City, 2012). Also, because the aim of community asset mapping is to locate resources, the interviewer must remember to ask participants for geographical information such as the addresses of resource locations (Healthy City, 2012). Typically, members of a community would not participate in interviews unless there are perceived benefits to participation. Although there can be great future benefits for individuals affected by a successful health advocacy effort, such benefits may not be motivating enough for people to participate in interviews because the benefits are not immediately apparent. Thus, an advocacy team may consider more obvious benefits such as monetary incentives or gift cards to encourage participation in interviews. An advocacy team may approach houses or go to populated areas and ask members of the community if they would be willing to be interviewed. Interviews for community asset mapping should be relatively short (about five to ten minutes), and can take place at the doorstep of houses or when standing at a public place. Interviewers also may provide a map if necessary to assist participants in locating community resources.

Surveys

An advocacy team also may use surveys to do community asset mapping (Healthy City, 2012). Surveys involve using a series of short questions to understand the perspectives of a respondent (see Guest et al., 2013). For example, to understand the perspectives of respondents regarding the need for more cancer-treatment facilities within a community, a survey may ask relevant questions such as whether more cancer-treatment facilities are necessary or not. If a majority of respondents indicate that more cancer-treatment facilities are necessary, the responses may reflect that the community may need more cancer-treatment facilities. There are various ways to conduct surveys, including face-to-face, telephone, or email. The survey approach largely depends on who the potential respondents are and what approach would be most suitable for them. For instance, if members of a community do not have high literacy rates, written surveys may not be suitable and face-to-face or telephone approaches may be better (Healthy City, 2012). Below is an example of what a survey question may look like:

1. How necessary is it for the community to have more cancer-treatment facilities? (please circle)

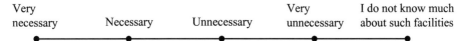

| Very necessary | Necessary | Unnecessary | Very unnecessary | I do not know much about such facilities |

According to Krosnick (1999), points on the rating scale should be labeled with words instead of numbers because words clarify the meaning of the scale points and can maximize validity. Krosnick also recommended that a survey should not have too many questions or else respondents may experience fatigue and consequently give perfunctory responses. An advocacy team should design a survey that is simple and clear for potential respondents to understand and avoid listing too many questions. For the purposes of community asset mapping for health advocacy, a survey with approximately twenty questions should suffice. Surveys may be effective for community asset mapping only in limited situations. Surveys may be useful if an advocacy team wants to determine that a certain resource is lacking within a community and that members of the community need more of that resource. Surveys also can be useful if an advocacy team already knows a few locations but wants the opinions of members in a community regarding the best location. For example, an advocacy team may already know that there are networking resources in towns A, B, and C, but the team may not know which town has the most networks and which town's networks are most relevant for the advocacy effort. In such a situation, surveys can inform the advocacy team regarding the best location because members of the community likely are more familiar with the community. In contrast, surveys may not be effective for community asset mapping if an advocacy team has very little idea about the community and its resource locations. For instance, an advocacy team may pick several locations at random and ask respondents to pick the optimal location, but doing so limits the answer to those provided as options on the survey. Below is an example of this limitation:

2. Which location in the community is most populated? (please circle)

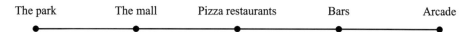

The park   The mall   Pizza restaurants   Bars   Arcade

As illustrated in the example, a respondent may be limited only to the five listed options, even though there may be other locations where there may be more people. A survey may insert an "others: please specify" option in the question so that respondents may provide an answer that is not listed among the available options. However, there may be a risk that the available options will influence the way a respondent thinks about another possible answer. For instance, the survey question above may cause a respondent to frame the idea of a populated location as a social or fun place, although other locations such as a factory or boot camp may be highly populated too. Also, having an "others: please specify" option may not be effective because respondents who are tired or unmotivated may choose one of the available options instead of putting in the effort to think of another possible answer. Decision-making that involves giving satisfactory answers instead of optimal and elaborately-thought-out answers is known as satisficing (Krosnick, 1999). Tired or unmotivated respondents may satisfice weakly and choose the available options instead of going through the effort of recalling the geographical layout of the community, thinking about which other locations might be more populated, comparing those locations with those listed in the survey, deciding the best location, and revising the decision process in order to be confident that the location was indeed the best. Because of the limitations of surveys for community asset mapping, an advocacy team should use surveys only in specific situations, particularly when the team already has some knowledge of the community.

Another approach to community asset mapping is to conduct community walks. Community walks can be a fun and practical way to conduct community asset mapping as they involve walking around the community to gain firsthand understanding of the community's layout and resource locations (Healthy City, 2012). An advocacy team may also interview members of the community as the team travels around the community. The team should carry with them a small map of the community during the walk as it can be useful for mapping out resources efficiently. Although community walks can be fun while allowing an advocacy team firsthand experience and understanding of the community's layout and resource locations, community walks can be a physically demanding task, especially if the advocacy team has few members or if the community is very big. An advocacy team may divide the workload by assigning various team members to different locations, but even with such teamwork, the physical effort required to walk around still is more demanding than other approaches such as conducting focus groups or telephone surveys. Furthermore, community walks can be time-consuming and an advocacy team may need several days of community walks to have a comprehensive understanding of the community's layout and resource locations. Given these limitations, community walks should be conducted only if the community is relatively small or if the advocacy team has many members. An advocacy team also may conduct community walks in conjunction with other approaches such as interviews and surveys.

An advocacy team may use an online mapping tool to aid the community asset mapping process. An online mapping tool consists of mapping software that is available on the Internet (Healthy City, 2012). An advocacy team may find such tools on various websites including HealthyCity.org (www.healthycity.org) and Google (http://maps.google.com/maps). However, such tools may be too complex for some individuals and may not be necessary for the purposes of health advocacy. Furthermore, storing vital information into such tools may not be an effective or safe approach because certain communities may not have reliable Internet access. Overall, a simple but accurate map and a few colorful stickers or pens should suffice for the purposes of community asset mapping in health advocacy.

There are four approaches to community asset mapping: focus groups, interviews, surveys, and community walks (Healthy City, 2012). These approaches are effective, but should be used in appropriate situations. For example, if an advocacy team only has a few members and a community is very big, an advocacy team should not do community walks, but should use other approaches such as telephone surveys instead. Accordingly, an advocacy team needs to assess which approach is most relevant and appropriate for the team and its targeted community.

The Usefulness of Community Asset Mapping

Now that community asset mapping and its methods have been introduced and elaborated upon, it is important to understand precisely how mapping resources is useful for health advocacy. There are three ways in which community asset mapping is useful for health advocacy: first, it helps an advocacy team know where the best locations are for advocating within a community. Second, it helps an advocacy team know the networks of people and organizations within a community. Third, it enables an advocacy team to see what resources are available or lacking within a community.

When an advocacy team successfully maps out the layout and resource locations of a community, the team is able to identify which location is most strategic for advocating purposes. For example, an advocacy team that wants to promote awareness about its campaign can use a community asset map to locate the most crowded area in a community. If an advocacy team wants to communicate with a specific audience, a community asset map also may help the team locate that audience. For instance, if an advocacy team wants to communicate to the elderly, a detailed community asset map can show where the community homes for elderly people are located. A community asset map is useful for strategic planning because it is able to categorize resources in a community. For example, the map can categorize crowded areas into groups that are more likely to have youths, working adults, or elderly people. With such categories, an advocacy team may strategically plan out the team's advocacy effort by focusing on relevant categories.

Community asset mapping also can help an advocacy team know the networks of people and organizations within a community. For example, a community asset map can be used to see who is involved in the network of a coalition. Again, a coalition is an alliance of people from various organizations who work together toward a shared goal (Sabatier, 1988; see also Weible et al., 2011). For example, a cancer coalition in a community may have partner organizations such as hospitals, clinics, social groups, schools, and churches within the same community to collaborate on cancer prevention and/or cancer treatment. If an advocacy team manages to persuade the cancer coalition to support the advocacy effort, the team may request that the coalition inform its partner organizations about the advocacy effort so that the team can focus on informing people and organizations outside of the coalition network. This kind of collaboration is very effective because the workload of promoting awareness is shared. Instead of investing time and effort to inform many organizations such as hospitals, clinics, social groups, schools, and churches, the advocacy team only needs to inform the cancer coalition organization. A community asset map also can help an advocacy team identify people and organizations outside the coalition network so that those outside the network may be reached effectively.

A community asset map enables an advocacy team to see what resources are available or lacking within a community. For instance, a community asset map may show the locations of various coalitions within a community. A coalition can be a valuable resource because of its expansive network. An advocacy team that knows the locations of various coalitions may choose the most beneficial and relevant for its advocacy effort. Without a community asset map, the advocacy team may not know which coalition would be most beneficial and relevant for the advocacy effort. Worse, the team may compromise and collaborate with a coalition that is unsuitable for the advocacy campaign. A community asset map also enables an advocacy team to identify resources that are lacking within a community. For instance, if a community asset map reveals that there are no coalitions within a community, the advocacy team may need to use a different approach to communicate the advocacy effort to numerous audiences in an efficient manner. In such a scenario, one possible alternative would be to persuade the media to relay the advocacy message to a mass audience. A community asset map also may help an advocacy effort if the map shows that resources are lacking. For instance, if the advocacy team is advocating for the allocation of more state resources into building cancer-treatment facilities, a community asset map that reveals few or no cancer-treatment facilities within the community can help reinforce the team's advocacy goal. Whether a community asset map shows that resources are available or lacking, an advocacy team can use the map to the team's advantage.

Key Informant Interviews

Another needs assessment method is conducting key informant interviews. Key informant interviews involve identifying and interviewing key individuals within a community (Marshall, 1996; Mattson & Hall, 2011). These key individuals often have significant influence on the way a health issue is addressed within a community. For example, if an advocacy team is advocating for more cancer-treatment facilities, a key informant may be the director of a cancer coalition within the community. Key informants are able to provide insightful information and can help an advocacy team to determine if there is a demand for health policy change. However, key informants may have opinions that are not reflective of what other members of the community perceive (Marshall, 1996). An advocacy team should conduct key informant interviews to understand the demand for health policy change and for enhancing the persuasiveness of advocacy messages, but the team should be mindful of responses from informants that are not reflective of the opinions of members within a community.

Key informant interviews can help an advocacy team ascertain if there is a demand for health policy change. For example, the director of a cancer coalition within a community may provide details about the progress or lack of progress in cancer treatment within the community. An advocacy team may be more confident about the need for health advocacy if key informants say there is a health issue that is not yet resolved. In contrast, if key informants say that there are adequate resources to manage a certain health issue and that change in health policy is not necessary, the advocacy team may need to reconsider proceeding with an advocacy effort. Key informants can be useful for needs assessment because they often have much experience in managing a health issue. For instance, the director of a cancer coalition may have years of experience in managing cancer in a community and may have substantial knowledge of the resources, support, funding, and networks available for cancer treatment within the community. Therefore, such key informants who are familiar with managing a health issue may provide the best assessments regarding the need for health policy change. Key informant interviews also can be useful for a needs assessment because it can save time for an advocacy team. Instead of interviewing many cancer patients, an advocacy team may be able to gauge the need for health policy change by interviewing a few key informants. However, interviewing a few key informants instead of patients should only be used in very limited circumstances, such as if the advocacy team has an impending deadline and has very little time remaining for advocacy. In most situations, key informant interviews should be conducted in conjunction with interviews with patients or individuals affected by the health issue.

The responses from key informant interviews may help enhance the persuasiveness of advocacy messages. When a key informant agrees that health policy change is necessary to address a health issue, an advocacy team may incorporate interview responses as supporting evidence for an advocacy argument in messages. For instance, if the director of a cancer coalition agrees that health policy change is necessary to address the lack of cancer-treatment facilities within a community, an advocacy team may use the response of the director as a credible supporting argument for the team's advocacy messages. Because the response came from an individual with a significant reputation and credibility within the community (i.e., director of a cancer coalition), the response can help make advocacy messages more persuasive (Petty, Cacioppo, & Goldman, 1981; see also Wathen & Burkell, 2002). An advocacy team may video record the interview session with a key informant and edit the recording afterwards so that it may be incorporated into advocacy messages. However, the advocacy team must first obtain permission from the key informant to video record the interview session, to edit the video, and to include the edited video into advocacy messages. Besides video recording, the advocacy team may do audio recording or transcribe key points from the interview. Some key informants may ignore an interview request or decline to be interviewed because of their status within an organization. An advocacy team should develop persuasive messages in order to get the attention of key informants and convince the informants to participate in interviews. Chapter 6 discusses strategies which an advocacy team can use to develop such persuasive messages.

Sometimes, the opinions of key informants may not be reflective of what other members of the community perceive (Marshall, 1996). For example, cancer patients in a community may say that there are insufficient cancer-treatment options available, but the director of a cancer coalition may claim otherwise. One reason for the differing of opinions may be because key informants may not share the same experiences as members in the community. For instance, the director of a cancer coalition may introduce many treatment options for cancer patients within a community, but the cancer patients may find those treatment options ineffective or unaffordable. Thus, the former may report that there are adequate cancer-treatment options, but the latter may think otherwise. Key informants also may feel threatened by an issue and thus differ in opinion. For example, the director of a coalition may not admit to a lack of cancer-treatment options because admitting may seem like conceding failure on the part of the coalition. Thus, in order to protect themselves, key informants might deny that an issue exists because admission may jeopardize their position. Therefore, an advocacy team should not merely interview key informants, but also should interview members of a community, too. Also, an advocacy team may interview different key informants to determine the legitimacy or accuracy of key informant claims. For example, an advocacy team may interview different key informants such as the founder of a club that supports cancer patients or the manager of a hospital and compare responses with those from the director of a cancer coalition. If the responses are similar, an advocacy team can have greater confidence that there is legitimacy to the claims of the key informants.

Conducting key informant interviews is an important procedure in needs assessment because key informants have significant insight into and experience with the advocated health issue within a community. The responses from key informant interviews can help an advocacy team determine whether there is a demand for health policy change. Also, if informants agree to support the advocacy team, the responses from informants may be incorporated into advocacy messages to enhance credibility and persuasiveness of advocacy messages. Key informant interviews should be conducted in conjunction with interviews with other members of the community to ensure accuracy of responses.

Summary

It is necessary for an advocacy team to do needs assessment because a health advocacy effort may not always be feasible or required. An advocacy team may not be able to launch an advocacy effort if the team has too many weaknesses or if there are too many external obstacles. An advocacy team may conduct a SWOT analysis in order to determine the strengths and weaknesses of the team and the external factors that may help or impede an advocacy effort. An advocacy team should launch an advocacy effort only when the SWOT analysis shows that the team has an adequate number of strengths and external factors that are helpful to the advocacy effort. An advocacy team also should know the layout of its targeted community well, including the location of important resources so those resources may be used effectively to the team's advantage. An advocacy team may use a community asset mapping technique to understand the layout of a community and to know the location of its resources. The four approaches that can be used to conduct community asset mapping include focus groups, interviews, surveys, and community walks. An advocacy team should choose an approach that will be most useful and appropriate for the team and its targeted community. Another procedure in needs assessment is the conducting of key informant interviews. Key informants can provide insightful responses and their experiences with the advocated health issue may help an advocacy team ascertain whether there is a need for an advocacy effort within the community. Furthermore, key informants often are people with significant reputation and credibility within the community, and their responses may be incorporated into advocacy messages to enhance the persuasiveness of the messages. The three procedures of SWOT analysis, community asset mapping, and key informant interviews can help an advocacy team determine if it is possible to conduct an advocacy campaign, if there is a problem that can be resolved by policy change, and if there is a demand for that change. After an advocacy team has determined that an advocacy effort is feasible and necessary, the team moves on to strategic planning.

References

DiCicco-Bloom, B., & Crabtree, B. F. (2006). The qualitative research interview. *Medical Education*, 40(4), 314–321. doi: 10.1111/j.1365-2929.2006.02418.x

Ebbeling, C. B., Pawlak, D. B., & Ludwig, D. S. (2002). Childhood obesity: Public-health crisis, common sense cure. *The Lancet*, 360(9331), 473–482. doi: 10.1016/S0140-6736(02)09678-2

Gregrich, R. J. (2003). A note to researchers: Communicating science to policy makers and practitioners. *Journal of Substance Abuse Treatment*, 25(3), 233–237. doi: 10.1016/S0740-5472(03)00120-X

Griffin, D., & Farris, A. (2010). School counselors and collaboration: Finding resources through community asset mapping. *Professional School Counseling*, 13(5), 248–256. doi: 10.5330/PSC.n.2010-13.248

Guest, G., Namey, E. E., & Mitchell, M. L. (2013). *Collecting qualitative data: A field manual for applied research*. Thousand Oaks, CA: Sage.

Healthy City. (2012). Participatory asset mapping: A community research lab toolkit. Burns, J. C., Pudrzynska Paul, D., & Paz, S. R. Retrieved from http://www.healthycity.org/

Krosnick, J. A. (1999). Survey research. *Annual Review of Psychology*, 50(1), 537–567. doi: 10.1146/annurev.psych.50.1.537

Lindlof, T.R., & Taylor, B. C. (2011). *Qualitative communication research methods* (3rd ed.). Thousand Oaks, CA: Sage.

Marshall, M. N. (1996). The key informant technique. *Family Practice*, 13(1), 92–97. doi: 10.1093/fampra/13.1.92

Mattson, M., & Hall, J. G. (2011). *Health as communication nexus*. Dubuque, IA: Kendall Hunt.

Petty, R. E., Cacioppo, J. T., & Goldman, R. (1981). Personal involvement as a determinant of argument-based persuasion. *Journal of Personality and Social Psychology*, 41(5), 847–855. doi:10.1037/0022-3514.41.5.847

Sabatier, P. A. (1988). An advocacy coalition framework of policy change and the role of policy-oriented learning therein. *Policy Sciences*, 21(2–3), 129–168. doi: 10.1007/BF00136406

Swinburn, B. A., Sacks, G., Hall, K. D., McPherson, K., Finegood, D. T., Moodie, M. L., & Gortmaker, S. L. (2011). The global obesity pandemic: Shaped by global drivers and local environments. *The Lancet*, *378*(9793), 804–814. doi: 10.1016/S0140–6736(11)60813–1

Wathen, C. N., & Burkell, J. (2002). Believe it or not: Factors influencing credibility on the Web. *Journal of the American Society for Information Science and Technology*, *53*(2), 134–144. doi: 10.1002/asi.10016

Weible, C. M., Sabatier, P. A., Jenkins-Smith, H. C., Nohrstedt, D., Henry, A., & deLeon, P. (2011). A quarter century of the advocacy coalition framework: An introduction to the special issue. *Policy Studies Journal*, *39*(3), 349–360. doi:10.1111/j.1541–0072.2011.00412.x

· 5 ·

FORMATIVE RESEARCH

After an advocacy team completes a needs assessment and ascertains that a particular health concern warrants an advocacy effort, the team proceeds to the formative research phase. In this phase, an advocacy team must gather statistical and related evidence that will inform the team about the advocated health issue. Also, the advocacy team must determine who its target audiences are. If this phase is executed well, an advocacy team will be able to craft more relevant advocacy messages because the team will have a better understanding of their target audiences and the advocated health issue. Also, due to its understanding of the target audiences, the advocacy team will be in a better position to anticipate possible reactions from target audience members.

Statistics

Formative research begins with gathering statistical information regarding the advocated health issue. An advocacy team needs to collect statistical evidence that will address three aspects of the advocated health issue: the prevalence, problems, and forecast of the health issue. First, documenting the prevalence of the health issue aids people in comprehending how big a problem is. For example, the United States was projected to have 1,660,290 new cancer cases and 580,350 cancer deaths in 2013 (Siegel, Naishadham, & Jemal, 2013). This alarming figure certainly will capture the attention of some audiences as these statistics are significant. Also, an advocacy team that is advocating for a cancer-related issue must have a thorough understanding of what it is that they are advocating for, thus knowing such statistical information is necessary. In some cases, the prevalence figure for a particular health concern may not be very high. Consequently, an advocacy team may not want to emphasize the low prevalence in their advocacy messages. Rather, the team only should mention the prevalence when asked or provide it as supplementary informa-tion during presentations. Although global or national prevalence statistics for a health issue are useful, an advocacy team also should collect prevalence data specific to the district or state in which the advocacy team is campaigning. Federal, district, and state prevalence data sometimes are unobtainable, but when there is such information, an advocacy team should collect that data because more local statistics will be more relevant for the campaign and its audiences.

It likely is not feasible for an advocacy team to measure prevalence; such an extensive and costly procedure is usually performed by researchers. Instead, an advocacy team should collect prevalence data either from a related health-care organization's website, through a search engine such as Google, or via another reliable source. For example, an advocacy team that is advocating for prosthetic parity may go to the Amputee Coalition's website, www.amputee-coalition.org, to find out the prevalence of amputees. Oftentimes such information can be found by clicking on the resources tab on the homepage of a healthcare organization's website. The other approach to find prevalence data is to use a search engine such as Google. Specifically, this book recommends using Google Scholar as it is easy to use and most often provides accurate and credible links to sources which contain appropriate information. However, most sources found through Google Scholar are academic journals which may require payment for access to articles. Although the cost for an article usually is not expensive, an advocacy team may decide against such spending. Instead an advocacy team may want to refer to the website of a reputable and related healthcare organization for statistical evidence as previously described.

Second, an advocacy team needs to collect statistical evidence that highlights the problems associated with the advocated health issue. For instance, if an advocacy team is trying to make wearing of helmets by motorcyclists a law within a state, the team should collect statistical evidences illustrating the problems motorcyclists can have when a helmet is not worn. For example, an advocacy team may find research evidence that motorcycle helmets reduce the likelihood of fatality in a crash by 37% (National Highway Traffic Safety Administration, 2005). An advocacy team needs to use such statistical evidence because doing so would make their advocacy arguments more compelling and persuasive. On the other hand, not using statistical evidence may compromise the credibility and persuasiveness of an advocacy team's arguments. As an illustration, compare these two claims below:

A: *Many motorcyclists die in accidents because they do not wear helmets.*

B: *In 2010, there were 4,502 motorcyclists who were killed in motorcycle crashes, and 709 of these motorcyclists may have been saved if they had worn helmets (Centers for Disease Control and Prevention, 2012)*

Which claim was more compelling? Because claim A has many deficits and claim B has greater substance, claim B is likely the more compelling claim. An advocacy team that uses claim A will not seem convincing because the claim is not specific, does not have a chronological reference, and has a misleading conclusion. Claim A is not specific when it mentions that "many motorcyclists die" because the exact number of motorcyclists is not given. Consequently, audiences who are told this claim may not understand the seriousness of not wearing a motorcycle helmet. Some audiences may think that "many motorcyclists" means 500 although the actual figure is more likely to be around 4,000 (see Centers for Disease Control and Prevention, 2012). Thus, having statistical information for a claim is important as it allows audiences to better comprehend the magnitude of a claim. Also, claim A does not give a chronological reference and therefore it is not known which year or years the information pertains to. Did many motorcyclists die in accidents since 2014? Or did many motorcyclists die in accidents in 1990? If audiences perceive the claim to mean the latter, these audiences may not feel impacted by the claim because 1990 may seem in the distant past and irrelevant to motorcycle safety in the present. Therefore, an advocacy team must use claims that are specific, so that audiences do not make inaccurate guesses stemming from ambiguity.

Claim A also has a misleading conclusion when "*because* they do not wear helmets" is mentioned. This conclusion seems to imply that the consequence of not wearing a helmet is fatality. However that is not always the case. There are many motorcyclists who are killed in accidents because of reasons other than not wearing helmets. For example, there have been motorcyclists who were killed in motorcycle crashes due to alcohol consumption and the reckless driving of other drivers on the road. The conclusion of claim A also is misleading because it can give the impression that wearing a helmet guarantees survival. However, this is not true; many motorcyclists who wear helmets also encounter fatal crashes. Furthermore, there can be fatal injuries to the body other than the head, and in such situations neither wearing a helmet nor not wearing a helmet would prevent fatality. A conclusion that would be clearer for claim A may be "Many motorcyclists died in accidents *but wearing helmets may have prevented many of the fatalities.*" Because claim A is not specific, does not have a chronological reference, and has a misleading conclusion, claim A cannot be considered good evidence for making advocacy arguments persuasive.

In contrast, claim B is more compelling because it is specific, has a chronological reference, and has an impactful and clear conclusion. Instead of using ambiguous terms such as "many," claim B gives precise numbers such as "4,502 motorcyclists who were killed in motorcycle crashes." Claim B also provides a chronological reference by mentioning that the year in which the accidents occurred was 2010. Also, claim B has an impactful conclusion as it alludes to the possibility that lives could have been saved if the motorcyclists wore helmets during the accidents. The conclusion of claim B is clear and it is based on research findings from the Centers for Disease Control and Prevention. Also, claim B's conclusion avoided definitive terms such as "because" or "would have." Instead, claim B mentioned that "709 motorcyclists *may* have been saved." The statistical evidence made claim B specific, relevant, and impactful, and therefore claim B is superior to claim A. In application, an advocacy team should find statistical evidence that addresses the problems of a health concern so that advocacy arguments are more compelling.

Third, an advocacy team should collect statistical evidence that provides a forecast of the health issue. A forecast can be useful in two ways: (1) it can illustrate how the health concern would continue to be a problem if it is not resolved by policy change; (2) it can show that there is a need for policy change. An example of the former is a forecast which shows the projected number of fatal motorcycle accidents in the future if helmet laws are not enforced. Such information can help the audiences of an advocacy team to conceptualize the detrimental consequence of not supporting the advocacy effort, and may thus motivate audiences to support the advocacy campaign. A forecast also can be used to show that there is a need for policy change. As an example, if an advocacy team is campaigning for a state to allocate more resources toward building cancer-treatment facilities, the team can show that change in resource allocation is necessary by presenting a forecast that cancer prevalence will increase by 75% over the next two decades (see Augustine, 2014). Such alarming projections may help a cancer-related advocacy campaign convince audiences that policy change is necessary. Sometimes, there may not be a forecast available for certain health concerns. This may occur because a health concern is relatively new and research is in early stages. In such situations, an advocacy team should not speculate as the team's credibility may be diminished if their speculations are unfounded. Instead, an advocacy team should focus on available statistical evidence that addresses prevalence and problems associated with the health issue, and use that evidence to persuade audiences that policy change is needed.

An advocacy team that uses statistical evidence can impress its audiences because the team appears to be credible, informed, and certain about its advocacy goal. In particular, an advocacy team should collect statistical evidence that addresses the prevalence, problems, and forecast of the advocated health issue. An advocacy team that incorporates this evidence into its advocacy messages may better compel and persuade its audiences to support the advocacy campaign.

Target Audiences

It is imperative that an advocacy team knows who its audiences are and understands the needs and preferences of the audiences. Failure to do so may lead to poor and uninformed development of advocacy messages, and the resulting messages that are disseminated may be deemed as inappropriate, irrelevant, or unimportant to audiences. When audiences respond undesirably to poorly designed messages, the advocacy effort may be in jeopardy because an advocacy effort hinges on the support of its audiences. Therefore, it is essential for an advocacy team to understand what is appropriate, relevant, and important for its audiences. Also, an advocacy team has to ascertain the audiences' level of awareness for the health issue and determine how much its audiences know or do not know about the advocated health issue. There usually are three primary audiences for health advocacy efforts: legislators, people directly or indirectly affected by the advocated health issue, and the media.

Legislators

Legislators are politicians in charge of specific districts or states who have a hand in creating and implementing policy (Bernheim, Rangel, & Rayo, 2006).

Because legislators are influential in making policy changes, their support for an advocacy effort is crucial. An advocacy team must consider what might be appropriate, relevant, and important for legislators so that the team develops effective advocacy messages. Because legislators often have very busy schedules, time is an important factor for them, and disseminating advocacy messages to legislators during irregular times might be inappropriate. For instance, Gregrich (2003) suggested that legislators are most busy during the start of a legislative session or budget cycle. Accordingly, an advocacy team must know when the opportune time is to communicate with legislators, so that the legislators may be most attentive and may not disregard the advocacy messages. Although legislators' schedules likely are not made public, a lobbyist may be able to inquire and find out when certain legislators are most available. There may be legislators who claim that they are always busy and thus cannot attend to the requests of an advocacy team. However, when an issue is significant and pressing, most legislators likely will attend to the issue or make time for the advocates. Thus, an advocacy team must consider what kinds of issues might be relevant and important enough to legislators to warrant their attention. The issues that are important to legislators often are tied to the issues that are important to their constituents. That is to say, because legislators are working for the welfare of residents in their districts or states, legislators often respond to the demands of their constituents. For example, if building more cancer-treatment facilities is important to state residents and they voice this concern to legislators, the legislators likely will have to lend an ear to what state residents are saying and consider if more resources should be allocated to building more cancer-treatment facilities. Ordinarily, state residents do not voice their concerns regarding health issues in unison; therefore, the onus of responsibility is on an advocacy team to inform, organize, persuade, and lead state residents to ask legislators for change. An advocacy team can do this in several ways, including getting district or state residents to sign a petition or attend a rally (discussed in Chapter 7). An advocacy team must emphasize in their advocacy messages to legislators that the advocated health issue is important to many district or state residents. Doing so may cause legislators to regard the health advocacy goals and related messages as more relevant and important.

An advocacy team must also ascertain the level of awareness that legislators have for the advocated health issue. For example, if an advocacy team is campaigning for more cancer-treatment facilities, the team must determine how much legislators know about cancer and cancer-treatment facilities. It is important to know the level of awareness that legislators have for an advocated health issue because advocacy messages have to be altered according to how much legislators know or do not know. For instance, if legislators are not very informed about cancer, an advocacy team may need to avoid using cancer-related jargon or terminology when communicating with legislators. Also, the advocacy team has to strategize and develop effective messages that explain important details about cancer in a succinct but clear way to legislators, so that legislators are not confused or stultified. On the other hand, if legislators have great knowledge about a health issue such as cancer, an advocacy team must work on collecting statistical evidence regarding cancer and become thoroughly familiar with the subject matter. By doing so, the team can be on par with legislators when communicating the advocacy message and be prepared for possible responses by legislators. A lobbyist may be helpful in finding out the level of awareness that legislators have regarding the advocated health issue. Through networks or personal communication, a lobbyist may be able to ascertain how much legislators know or do not know and report to the advocacy team the level of awareness legislators have so that the team can strategize accordingly.

Relevant Populations

The relevant populations that an advocacy team must know and understand are people who are affected directly or indirectly by the advocated health issue. For example, if an advocacy team is campaigning for legislation to restrict food marketing that targets children (see Ebbeling, Pawlak, & Ludwig, 2002; Swinburn et al., 2011), people directly affected by the food marketing are children and people indirectly affected may be parents. Because the people who are directly and indirectly affected experience the health issue differently, the two groups will be examined separately.

Most often, people who are experiencing the health issue themselves are the people most directly affected by the health issue. Examples include cancer patients, amputees, the visually impaired, and so on. Thus, a directly affected population often is the most supportive of an advocacy effort because they can most directly benefit from a successful advocacy campaign. At the same time, a directly affected population experiences the consequences of the health issue most and therefore may be unable to support advocacy to the fullest. For instance, cancer patients going through chemotherapy experience much fatigue (Goedendorp et al., 2012) and therefore may not be in a condition to support an advocacy effort such as attending a rally. Sometimes, persuading such patients to support in ways that may not require much physical effort (e.g., online petition) also can be a daunting task because these patients may not be in a good emotional state or are too burdened with the health issue. Therefore, although a directly affected population may be most supportive of an advocacy effort, they may not be in a condition to directly support the advocacy effort. Accordingly, an advocacy team must understand and ascertain what is relevant and important for a directly affected population while considering what is appropriate as well.

Often, anything that helps a directly affected population with their health issue is relevant and important to them. However, some forms of help may be perceived as more important or urgently required than other forms of assistance. For instance, amputees may regard prosthetic parity as more important than the building of accessible infrastructure for the disabled in communities. Although both are important, prosthetic parity takes precedence over building of accessible infrastructure and the former may be needed first; if amputees cannot afford prosthetic limbs, they may not travel independently and use accessible infrastructure. An advocacy team needs to know what is most important to a directly-affected population and cater to that population's needs. One approach that an advocacy team may use to find out what is regarded as most important to the directly affected population is to conduct focus groups. A focus group session in this context involves recruiting members of the directly-affected population to participate in a group interview session. Through this session, an advocacy representative conducts the interview to ask and understand what concern is most pertinent to the directly affected population (Chapter 7 discusses focus groups in greater length). However, members of a directly-affected population may not be willing or able to participate in a focus group session. For example, some cancer patients may be experiencing fatigue or may be burdened by the disease and decide not to participate in a focus group session. In such situations, an advocacy team may conduct focus group sessions with the families, close friends, or caregivers of people who are directly affected by the advocated health issue.

An advocacy team must also determine what is considered appropriate for a directly-affected population. Sometimes, a directly affected population can be sensitive to matters concerning the health issue, and thus unvarnished communication about the health issue to a directly-affected population may be inappropriate. For instance, cancer patients already know the negative aspects of the disease, and therefore highlighting those negative aspects in advocacy messages is inappropriate as the messages may only serve to further burden the cancer patients. An advocacy team also may conduct focus groups with members of a directly-affected population to determine what may be appropriate or inappropriate. In the event that members of the directly-affected population cannot or are unwilling to participate in focus group sessions, an advocacy team may approach the families, close friends, or caregivers of the people directly affected by the health issue.

In some cases, an advocacy team may need to be forthright about the health issue because it would be the appropriate thing to do. For instance, children who are targeted by food marketing (see Ebbeling et al., 2002; Swinburn et al., 2011) are the directly-affected population, but they may not know that they are being targeted. Also, children may not know how targeted food marketing can be harmful to them. In such cases, an advocacy team has to be straightforward in describing the harm of targeted food marketing to children. Because the directly-affected population in this instance is children, it may be inappropriate to use difficult terms, jargon, or challenging statistical illustrations in communication with them. Thus, not only is appropriateness dependent on what the health issue is, appropriateness also is dependent on the age of the audiences. As another example, if an advocacy team is campaigning for more elder-care facilities to be built and the directly-affected population is the elderly, it may be inappropriate to communicate to the elderly in advanced technological terms and jargon as the elderly may not be familiar with such technology or jargon. For instance, because the elderly may not be proficient in using the Internet or social media, an advocacy team may not be successful with its efforts if it requests that the elderly sign online petitions or support the advocacy effort by "liking" the team's Facebook page.

Another factor that influences appropriateness is culture. What may be considered appropriate in one culture may be deemed inappropriate in another culture. For example, an advocacy message that stresses the consequences of nonparticipation may cause a cultural group to support the advocacy effort, but a Hispanic audience may not respond well to the advocacy message as it may be too confrontational for them (see Huerta & Macario, 1999). Accordingly, an advocacy team should recognize the cultural expectations for a directly-affected population and avoid violating the cultural norms. To establish what is appropriate, an advocacy team must determine how sensitive the advocated health issue is, the age group, and culture of the directly affected population.

Most, if not all, people directly affected by an advocated health issue have great level of awareness about the health issue. For example, an amputee who cannot afford a prosthetic limb already knows how difficult it is to manage without a prosthetic limb. Therefore, it is unnecessary for an advocacy team to extensively inform a directly-affected population about the health issue. As previously mentioned, there can be exceptions, such as a directly-affected population that is unaware of being affected by a health issue (e.g., children who are targeted by food marketing). An advocacy team needs to determine the directly-affected population's level of awareness about the health issue so that redundancy may be avoided or elaboration may be given in advocacy messages.

The people who are indirectly affected by the advocated health issue mostly are family members or caretakers of the directly affected population. Sometimes, people indirectly affected by the health issue can be very supportive of an advocacy effort not only because of their close ties with directly-affected people, but also because they too experience significant burdens providing care for the directly-affected persons. For example, family members can experience economical and psychological burdens in taking care of a family member with multiple sclerosis, including paying medical expenses and experiencing symptoms of depression or anxiety (Buhse, 2008). Because members of an indirectly-affected population may experience significant burdens, an advocacy team must be tactful in communicating with this population. An advocacy team should not appear indifferent to the burdens experienced by members of the indirectly-affected population.

Also, because people who are indirectly affected by the health issue usually have close ties with those who are directly affected, communicating about the health issue can be a sensitive topic and an advocacy team should be mindful of what is appropriate to communicate. Similar to a directly-affected population, an advocacy team may find out what is considered appropriate to an indirectly-affected population by conducting focus group sessions. Sometimes, an indirectly-affected population is more physically able to attend focus group sessions than a directly-affected population, since the former often is not restricted by the physical or emotional effects of a health issue. For example, family members of people with cancer may not experience the fatigue that people with cancer experience (see Goedendorp et al., 2012). However, there can be exceptions. For instance, certain health issues, such as multiple sclerosis, require much physical effort on the part of family members (Buhse, 2008) and therefore the indirectly-affected population may not be able to attend focus group sessions due to tiredness. In such situations, an advocacy team may approach the close friends or relatives of the family members for the focus group sessions.

Sometimes, members of an indirectly-affected population may be more physically able to attend focus group sessions, but they may not be willing to attend those sessions. This may occur because attending a focus group session may seem like a costly endeavor, especially for caregivers as they may have to invest much time and money taking care of someone (see Buhse, 2008). For instance, if a caregiver has to spend the majority of a day taking care of a person and can finally have time to rest, that caregiver may find the notion of resting more appealing than attending a focus group session because the former is rejuvenating, but the latter may be regarded as exhausting. As another example, a caretaker who spends much time taking care of a person may need the available time remaining to work for wages, and so attending a focus group session may seem to compromise that time allocated for earning wages. An advocacy team may decide in such situations to contact an indirectly-affected population by phone or email. However, the use of phone and email can be limiting because an advocacy team can only get one person's perspective through a phone call or an email message. An advocacy team may conduct multiple phone calls or use an email thread, but cross-comparing multiple responses can be arduous, inaccurate, and complex. Although the use of phone or email may not be as useful as a focus group session in understanding common experiences shared by many members in an indirectly-affected population, in some circumstances phone or email may be the only viable options. Therefore, understanding a population's perspective via phone or email should be used with caution.

Similar to people directly affected by a health issue, an indirectly-affected population likely will regard the advocated health issue as being relevant and important. As previously mentioned, the resources of time and money may be important to caregivers too, therefore an advocacy team may want to communicate to caregivers that supporting the advocacy effort is worth the investment of time and possible compromising of wages. If time is a resource that is important to an indirectly-affected population, an advocacy team must plan ways to address the issue of time in advocacy messages. For instance, if an indirectly-affected population is not confident that committing time to support an advocacy effort is worth it, an advocacy team may want to establish credibility with the indirectly-affected population. When an advocacy team appears credible and capable, an indirectly affected population may be more confident that investing time in supporting the advocacy effort will be worthwhile and will reap positive results. An advocacy team may communicate credibility by emphasizing that the team had been successful in previous advocacy efforts, or that the team is comprised of leading health experts and professionals, or that the team has the backing of the media (provided these are true claims).

If the concern is about foregoing earning wages in order to spend time to support an advocacy effort, an advocacy team may want to address the benefits of a successful advocacy effort so that the costs associated with not earning wages may seem worth it. For example, an advocacy team may communicate what the advocacy goal is and how it can positively benefit the caregivers and people experiencing the health issue. However, an advocacy team must be mindful not to promise things that it cannot be sure of delivering. For instance, an advocacy team must not guarantee that the legislature will pass a new law if people support the advocacy effort, because this result cannot be guaranteed. If an advocacy team makes claims that are later proved to be false, supporters may become disappointed and discouraged, and future advocacy efforts will be compromised because supporters may no longer trust such advocacy campaigns. Furthermore, an advocacy team may become embroiled in legal issues if a former supporter decides to press charges against the advocacy team for its false promises. Thus, an advocacy team can communicate the potential benefits of a successful advocacy campaign and the expectations of the campaign outcome, but an advocacy team must not make guarantees about the outcome. An advocacy team needs to ascertain what is regarded as important to an indirectly-affected population, including time and financial issues. However, time and money may not be the only concerns of an indirectly-affected population. Therefore, an advocacy team needs to assess what further concerns there may be in order to communicate the advocacy effort more effectively to target audiences. Again, an advocacy team may find out what the concerns are by conducting focus group sessions.

Similar to a directly-affected population, the level of awareness of the advocated health issue should be high for an indirectly-affected population. Therefore, an advocacy team may focus less on informing about the health issue and instead focus more on communicating what the advocacy effort may bring if it is successful and how people may support the advocacy effort. Often, an indirectly-affected population may be uncertain, even skeptical, about an advocacy effort. As previously mentioned, an advocacy team can circumvent the uncertainty or skepticism by emphasizing the team's credibility. The team can do so by highlighting the caliber of the advocacy team members or the team's advocacy success record (i.e., if the team has had previous successful advocacy experiences). An advocacy team should prepare any necessary statistical evidence or information that may be helpful in reducing uncertainties regarding the advocacy effort. Similar to a directly-affected population, sometimes an indirectly-affected population may not be aware that they are being affected indirectly by a health issue. For instance, parents might not be aware that their children are targeted by food marketing (see Ebbeling et al., 2002; Swinburn et al., 2011). In such situations, an advocacy team should elaborate on the health issue as well when communicating with an indirectly-affected population.

Relevant populations refer to the people who are directly and indirectly affected by the advocated health issue. Those who are indirectly affected by the health issue may share similar experiences with a directly-affected population, but there also are many contrasting experiences to consider. An advocacy team must cater to the two groups accordingly and plan advocacy messages that will be appropriate, relevant, important, and consistent with the relevant populations' level of awareness regarding the health issue.

The Media

The media refer to organizations that specialize in mass communication of information (e.g., news) through channels such as the radio, television, newspapers, and the Internet (e.g., Chyi, Yang, Lewis, & Zheng, 2010; Korda & Itani, 2013; Stryker, Moriarty, & Jensen, 2008; Rosales, 2013). Because most media companies are for-profit companies, profitability or viewership/listenership potential is the most appropriate, relevant, and important concern for these media companies. Therefore, an advocacy team will need to consider profitability and viewership/listenership potential in developing effective advocacy messages.

An advocacy team needs to consider how the media may profit from supporting an advocacy campaign. There are three possible ways: First, an advocacy team may pay a premium fee for having their campaign advertised on the radio or on television. However, such an approach can be costly (Farrelly, Hussin, & Bauer, 2007), and an advocacy team may want to consider the other two ways instead. Second, the media may benefit from enhanced public image for supporting a notable advocacy cause. An advocacy team may emphasize in advocacy messages that people may develop favorable opinions of media companies that support notable causes. Third, an advocacy team may offer to advertise a media company in exchange for being advertised on media. For example, an advocacy campaign may have information of a supporting media company in their advocacy pamphlets, banners, and so on. This is similar to a "sponsorship" deal.

These profitability concerns often pertain to media that do not specialize in news. An advocacy team may approach media that do not specialize in news such as a music radio station. However, news media may be the optimal channel for advocacy purposes. The news media are not only a more relevant channel for health advocacy, they also can help an advocacy campaign to appear more serious, urgent, and legitimate (Wallack & Dorfman, 1996). Although most news media also are for-profit, the manner in which they profit is different from other media outlets. Specifically, the news media profit from high viewership/listenership. Therefore, an advocacy team needs to consider how the advocacy campaign may have potential to garner high viewership/listenership.

Most media have sensationalistic approaches to covering news (see e.g., Caulfield & Bubela, 2004; Grabe, Zhou, & Barnett, 2001) and therefore an advocacy team should consider how the advocacy campaign may be suitable for news coverage. For example, an advocacy team may conduct a rally with signboards and banners outside a statehouse. Such an approach may be newsworthy for the media to report about. Also, an advocacy team should consider how the advocated health issue is relevant to the media's audiences. For example, prosthetic parity may not be an appealing issue for the news media to report about unless the advocacy team convinces the media that prosthetic parity is a concern of many of the media's audiences. News that is not relevant to the media's audiences likely is not reported, whereas relevant news more likely will be. An advocacy team should consider how the advocacy campaign may be appealing and relevant to the media's audiences.

It may be inappropriate to inundate the media with excessive information about the health advocacy campaign. Because most media are for-profit organizations, the media may be more interested in how they may benefit from supporting an advocacy campaign instead of other aspects of the campaign, such as the advocated health issue. Therefore, an advocacy team should be mindful not to provide superfluous information to the media. Excessive information may stultify the media and consequently dampen their interest for the advocacy campaign. Unless the media ask for more details, the advocacy team should focus on communicating profit-oriented concerns to the media. The media may likely ask for more details when they decide to support an advocacy campaign.

The media's level of awareness for an advocated health issue largely depends on how pertinent the health issue is for the community that the media are located in. For example, if the media are located in the state of Indiana, the advocated health issue concerns water sanitation, and water sanitation is a relevant issue that many residents in Indiana experience, then the media in Indiana likely have high awareness of the advocated health issue. This is because the media likely are informed about the happenings within the community that it extensively reports about. In contrast, if the health issue is excessive UV-light exposure and residents in Indiana do not identify with this problem, it is unlikely that the media in Indiana know much about the health issue. Whether the media's level of awareness for an advocated health issue is high or low, an advocacy team should not inform the media about the health issue at length unless the media make a request for more information. This is because an advocacy team should not inundate the media with excessive information and risk losing the interest of the media. However, if the media's level of awareness is high for an advocated health issue, it may be easier for an advocacy team to persuade the media to support the advocacy campaign because the campaign is likely pertinent to the media's audiences and therefore newsworthy.

An advocacy team needs to plan advocacy messages that will address profit concerns for the media. Particularly, an advocacy team needs to consider how the advocacy campaign is relevant and newsworthy for the media to report about. An advocacy team also should be mindful not to provide excessive information so that the media's interest in supporting the advocacy campaign won't be dampened.

Summary

After an advocacy team determines through needs assessment that an advocacy effort is warranted, the team will proceed with formative research. An advocacy team will have to collect statistical data that will inform the team about the advocated health issue. Specifically, the team should collect data regarding the prevalence, problems, and forecast of the health issue. After gathering statistical data, an advocacy team should identify target audiences and understand what is considered appropriate, relevant, and important to those audiences. Target audiences in the context of health advocacy often are composed of legislators, relevant populations, and the media. An advocacy team also should understand what level of awareness these target audiences have in regards to the advocated health issue. Understanding target audiences will allow an advocacy team to develop better advocacy messages and anticipate possible reactions of the target audiences. After an advocacy team has collected statistical data and identified target audiences, the advocacy team will proceed to the messaging process. The messaging process is discussed in the next chapter.

References

Augustine, P. (2014). Cancer in developing countries—concerns. *International Journal of Preventive and Therapeutic Medicine*, 2(1), 3–4. Retrieved from http://ijptm.com/index.php/ijptm

Bernheim, B. D., Rangel, A., & Rayo, L. (2006). The power of the last word in legislative policy making. *Econometrica*, 74(5), 1161–1190. doi: 10.1111/j.1468–0262.2006.00701.x

Buhse, M. (2008). Assessment of caregiver burden in families of persons with multiple sclerosis. *Journal of Neuroscience Nursing*, 40(1), 25–31. Retrieved from http://www.lww.com/

Caulfield, T., & Bubela, T. (2004). Media representations of genetic discoveries: Hype in the headlines? *Health Law Review*, 12(2), 53–61. Retrieved from http://www.hli.ualberta.ca/

Centers for Disease Control and Prevention (2012). Helmet use among motorcyclists who died in crashes and economic cost savings associated with state motorcycle helmet laws—United States, 2008–2010. *Morbidity and Mortality Weekly Report*, 61(23), 425–430. Retrieved from http://www.cdc.gov/

Chyi, H. I., Yang, M. J., Lewis, S. C., & Zheng, N. (2010). Use of and satisfaction with newspaper sites in the local market: Exploring differences between hybrid and online-only users. *Journalism & Mass Communication Quarterly*, 87(1), 62–83. doi: 10.1177/107769901008700104

Ebbeling, C. B., Pawlak, D. B., & Ludwig, D. S. (2002). Childhood obesity: Public-health crisis, common sense cure. *The Lancet*, 360(9331), 473–482. doi: 10.1016/S0140–6736(02)09678–2

Farrelly, M. C., Hussin, A., & Bauer, U. E. (2007). Effectiveness and cost effectiveness of television, radio and print advertisements in promoting the New York smokers' quitline. *Tobacco Control*, 16(Suppl 1), i21–i23. doi: 10.1136/tc.2007.019984

Goedendorp, M. M., Andrykowski, M. A., Donovan, K. A., Jim, H. S., Phillips, K. M., Small, B. J., ... & Jacobsen, P. B. (2012). Prolonged impact of chemotherapy on fatigue in breast cancer survivors. *Cancer*, 118(15), 3833–3841. doi: 10.1002/cncr.26226

Grabe, M., Zhou, S., & Barnett, B. (2001). Explicating sensationalism in television news: Content and the bells and whistles of form. *Journal of Broadcasting & Electronic Media*, 45(4), 635–655. doi: 10.1207/s15506878jobem4504_6

Gregrich, R. J. (2003). A note to researchers: Communicating science to policy makers and practitioners. *Journal of Substance Abuse Treatment, 25*(3), 233–237. doi: 10.1016/S0740-5472(03)00120-X

Huerta, E. E., & Macario, E. (1999). Communicating health risk to ethnic groups: Reaching Hispanics as a case study. *Journal of the National Cancer Institute Monographs, 1999*(25), 23–26. Retrieved from http://jncimono.oxfordjournals.org/

Korda, H., & Itani, Z. (2013). Harnessing social media for health promotion and behavior change. *Health Promotion Practice, 14*(1), 15–23. doi: 10.1177/1524839911405850

National Highway Traffic Safety Administration (2005). Traffic safety facts laws: Motorcycle helmet use laws. *National Center for Statistics and Analysis,* 1–4. Retrieved from http://www.nhtsa.gov/

Rosales, R. G. (2013). Citizen participation and the uses of mobile technology in radio broadcasting. *Telematics and Informatics, 30*(3), 252–257. doi: 10.1016/j.tele.2012.04.006

Siegel, R., Naishadham, D., & Jemal, A. (2013). Cancer statistics, 2013. *CA: A Cancer Journal for Clinicians, 63*(1), 11–30. doi: 10.3322/caac.21166

Stryker, J. E., Moriarty, C. M., & Jensen, J. D. (2008). Effects of newspaper coverage on public knowledge about modifiable cancer risks. *Health Communication, 23*(4), 380–390. doi: 10.1080/10410230802229894

Swinburn, B. A., Sacks, G., Hall, K. D., McPherson, K., Finegood, D. T., Moodie, M. L., & Gortmaker, S. L. (2011). The global obesity pandemic: Shaped by global drivers and local environments. *The Lancet, 378*(9793), 804–814. doi: 10.1016/S0140-6736(11)60813-1

Wallack, L., & Dorfman, L. (1996). Media advocacy: A strategy for advancing policy and promoting health. *Health Education & Behavior, 23*(3), 293–317. doi: 10.1177/109019819602300303

· 6 ·

MESSAGING PROCESS

The messaging process within the Health Communication Advocacy Model (Mattson, 2010) is crucial. It is the stage during which the team's position statement is translated into messages that are crafted to be as persuasive as possible in an effort to meet the team's advocacy goals. The aim is to design messages that are compelling enough to encourage target audiences to be in favor of the team's position statement on a health issue. This can be achieved if the team uses communication theories and concepts in developing its message. A caveat to note is that there are individual differences in receiving and responding to messages (Moore, Harris, & Chen, 1995; Venkatraman, Marlino, Kardes, & Sklar, 1990). However, the effects of communication concepts in message construction have been well documented (see e.g., Witte & Allen, 2000) and should be taken into account. In the messaging process stage, there are five key elements that an advocacy team must consider in crafting a message. The message needs to be: stimulating, motivational, eliminating barriers, culturally consistent, and within the resource capabilities of the organization.

Stimulating Messages

Messages should be simple, straightforward, and framed in a way that would be optimal for the audience to comprehend the relevance of the message to the health issue (Randolph & Viswanath, 2004). A message also should grab the audience's attention, and this can be done by arousing their emotions and through the use of visual and audio techniques.

Emotions

Messages that are emotionally stimulating may instigate change in audiences. For instance, studies have shown that fear-inducing messages have a greater propensity to invoke attitudinal and behavioral change in target audiences (Witte & Allen, 2000). The use of emotional appeals should be executed with care though, as inappropriate use of emotional appeals might result in backlash effects, such as audiences becoming offended or afraid because of the message (Guttman & Salmon, 2004). Common emotional appeals used in messages include fear, anger, and guilt appeals.

Fear appeals are persuasive communication efforts that aim to motivate preventive action and self-protective behaviors in audiences by triggering an unpleasant emotional state through presentation of threatening stimuli (Ruiter, Abraham, & Kok, 2001). The use of fear appeals should be coupled with high-efficacy messages in order to promote positive behavioral change (Witte & Allen, 2000). For example, when a campaign team decides to advocate for restricting the selling of cigarettes to adolescents, the team can depict images of possible detrimental consequences of chronic smoking, such as an illustration of deteriorating tissue due to lung cancer. However, there should be incorporated messages that provide audiences with a manageable solution, such as a brief description of what they can do to prevent such illnesses (in this case, it would be to join your team's cause and avoid smoking). Fear appeals can be effective, but only when coupled with a viable solution to the problem.

Anger is stirred by situations where either goal-oriented behavior is hindered by obstacles or when demeaning offences are perceived to be acted out against a person or a person's loved ones (Nabi, 1999). Anger appeals therefore communicate the possibility of such violations toward the audience. Anger appeals are useful for confronting issues, behaviors, or policies that restrict the rights of people (Turner, 2007). Nabi (1999) suggested that anger churns high levels of energy for the purpose of defending oneself or one's loved ones, or for resolving something deemed to be wrong. Messages that use anger appeals must be explicit and clear in showing how the audience's goals are threatened and that the problem can be resolved (Turner, 2007). Anger appeals are especially useful for attempts to change health policies or regulations, as a combination of anger and strong efficacy can produce the desired motivation in audiences that is necessary for supporting such efforts (Turner, 2012). As an example of effective use of anger appeals, an advocacy team might design a message illustrating the lack of health insurance coverage for people within a certain demographic (e.g., age, disability) and persuade the audience that the solution is for them to sign the team's petition. Anger appeals, just like any emotional appeal, may work only when used appropriately and in tandem with an efficacy component.

Guilt is the distress experienced when one realizes that a personally relevant social or moral standard has been violated (Kugler & Jones, 1992). Guilt appeals rely on highlighting the discrepancy between one's own conduct and personal standards, or between one's well-being and the well-being of other people (Coulter, Cotte, & Moore, 1999). The use of guilt appeals in persuasive messages is designed to elicit guilt in audiences and to present them with a recommended course of action to mitigate the guilt (O'Keefe, 2002). It is important to note that the use of guilt appeals is not suitable for audiences who are the victims of violation; rather, guilt appeals should be used with audiences whose violations affect others, but are controllable (Turner, 2012). For instance, an advocacy team may choose to communicate to a targeted audience that, unlike themselves, there are many people who are uninsured and cannot afford health insurance coverage (e.g., Dubay, Holahan, & Cook, 2007), and then prompt the audience to stand up against this inequality by signing a petition for change. Coulter et al. (1999) posited that guilt appeals are more likely to be effective if the message is perceived to be credible; on the contrary, if the source appears to be using inappropriate tactics to manipulate people, then audiences will react negatively and experience other emotions such as annoyance instead of guilt. As it is with other forms of emotional appeal, the use of guilt in messages has to be developed and performed with considerable care (Guttman & Salmon, 2004).

Visual and Audio Techniques

Messages that are more stimulating can be more effective. Stimulating messages can be achieved when messages incorporate visual and/or audio elements. For example, web browsers who viewed a testimonial ad that was in audio/video format were more likely to identify with the characters in the testimonial ad and be more favorable to the website than web browsers who viewed a text/picture testimonial ad (Appiah, 2006). In a study of television messages, Lang, Dhillon, and Dong, (1995) showed that arousing messages were remembered better than calm messages. Thus, stimulating messages may be more effective, and designing such messages can be accomplished through effective visual and/or audio techniques.

The use of visual elements in messages may be an effective tool for communicating advocacy efforts. For example, in one study, pictures that were rated as highly arousing were remembered better than pictures that were low in arousal ratings (Bradley, Greenwald, Petry, & Lang, 1992). The relationship between imagery and psychological processes has been well established in the literature. For instance, in a study examining people viewing and/or listening to a news presentation on a small screen, attention, knowledge acquisition, and memory were found to be enhanced when viewing a moving facial image presenting positive messages as opposed to a static facial image (Ravaja, 2004). In application, if advocacy teams desire to use communication channels such as videos posted on the Internet, it might be advantageous for the team to opt for designing videos with engaging and moving images rather than static illustrations. The use of vivid imagery can also be beneficial. According to Smith and Shaffer (2000), when a campaign message employs vivid imagery that is congruent with the theme of the message, it helps the audience process the message. This was determined to be particularly true for audiences who had low need for cognition and were not motivated to analyze the message. The notion of congruency deserves attention, as campaigns that use vivid images that are incongruent with the message will result in inhibition of message processing. For instance, if a campaign team is trying to garner support from affected populations in a health advocacy effort concerning human immuno-deficiency virus (HIV), but uses visual elements of teenage gang violence in its messages, the discrepancy would leave the audience puzzled and unable to process the message effectively. In this case, although imagery of teenage gang violence might be stimulating and startling, there is no real or direct relation to HIV. The use of congruent vivid imagery, however, helps enhance persuasion and message recall.

Messages also can be stimulating and effective when audio features are emphasized. According to Rodero (2012), the use of sound effects (i.e., sounds that depict situations or environments such as a car crash) and sound shots (i.e., changes in sound intensity to convey spatial distance such as a car crash far away) can enhance listener attention. Thus, in the message design process the advocacy campaign team might want to consider incorporating a combination of sound effects and sound shots. As was the case for visual imagery, stimulating sounds affect psychological processes as well. Bradley and Lang (2000) found that sounds that were highly arousing, whether pleasant or not, were remembered better than sounds with lower arousal ratings. Potter (2000) posited in a study of radio messages that with more voice actors/actresses in a message, the amount of processing resources allocated for encoding information in the audio message increases for the listener. In application, an advocacy team crafting a message should consider using multiple voice talents instead of just one voice actor/actress. Crucially too, the placement of information should be carefully managed, as information that is positioned immediately after a voice change is not processed as effectively as information given later on. That is, important details should not be presented immediately after (i.e., less than three seconds) a voice change (Potter, 2000). The use of sounds, like any other tool, should be incorporated appropriately, and negligent utilization of sounds can lead to adverse effects. For example, irrelevant sounds can interfere with memory (Banbury, Macken, Tremblay, & Jones, 2001). Thus, health advocacy teams need to be careful in incorporating sounds in designing messages.

By designing and implementing stimulating messages, advocacy teams put themselves in a better position to communicate their ideas for change and persuade their target audiences toward that change. Advocacy messages can be stimulating by using emotional appeals, visual elements, or audio techniques.

Motivational Messages

Although it is important for messages to be stimulating, it also is essential for messages to motivate audiences to engage in the desired response. This can be achieved through conveying to the audience their susceptibility to a threat and how it affects them, or by including self-disclosure in the message.

Audiences need to realize their vulnerability to a threatening health concern in order for them to consider action. When the perceived threat is low, audiences likely will be unmotivated to process advocacy messages further, and there will not be a response to the message (Witte, 1994). If an advocacy message does not illustrate that a health issue needs to be addressed or is pressing, audiences likely will be dismissive of the message and avoid involvement. Thus, the message needs to convey a high level of risk, communicating that audiences stand to be affected negatively if they do not take action. For example, advocacy messages might address to parents the notion that children are increasingly obese due to environmental factors such as fast food and food marketing directed at children (Ebbeling, Pawlak, & Ludwig, 2002; Swinburn et al., 2011). Such a message would alert parents as it stresses how such environmental factors may affect their children.

Although the threat level should be high in order to motivate the audience to process the message, it is imperative that solutions be presented to audiences to make them feel that there are means to resolve the threat by engaging in a recommended response. This is referred to as perceived efficacy. There are two forms of perceived efficacy: perceived response efficacy, which is the believed effectiveness of the recommended action to thwart the threat, and perceived self-efficacy, which is an individual's confidence to carry out the recommended action (Witte, 1992). According to Witte (1994), a combination of high levels of risk and high levels of efficacy results in an optimal amount of message acceptance. Thus, advocacy messages should incorporate efficacy as well, describing explicitly the recommended action for an audience to take along with how to confidently perform that action. Continuing with the aforementioned example about obesity in children, such an advocacy message should mention clearly the recommended action for parents to take, such as signing an online petition to advance the proposal for restricting food marketing directed at children. It is important to note that the prescribed efficacy message must be perceived to be effective and manageable to deal with the threat, or else the audience would cave into their fear associated with the threat (Witte, 1994). Witte (1991) further warned that regardless of efficacy level, if threat level is low, attitude, intention, and behavioral change will be low. Therefore, an advocacy team should be consistently mindful of the need for both threat level and efficacy level to be high, with the latter being presented and perceived as both effective and manageable.

Another method to motivate audiences to engage in the desired response is to include self-disclosure in the message. Han (2009) postulated that people are more inclined to be motivated to participate in a political appeal if the message includes self-disclosure. In Han's experiment, people who heard an appeal with disclosure of some personal information were twice as likely to make donations to a cause as participants who heard an appeal without the element of self-disclosure. This phenomenon resonates with the review done by Collins and Miller (1994), in which they reported that greater self-disclosure promotes liking. Health advocacy messages can effectively incorporate self-disclosure through the use of testimonials, which may be especially effective when emotional appeals and visual/audio techniques are incorporated.

Motivating audiences to perform the desired response of the advocacy message, such as signing petitions or contributing to campaigns, may be accomplished by relaying to the audiences the risks they are vulnerable to or by having self-disclosure in the message. In conveying risks, it is essential that an effective and manageable solution is provided. Self-disclosure, which promotes liking, can be done through testimonials. These methods may be useful in instigating audiences to take action.

Eliminate Barriers

Advocacy messages should eliminate barriers that may hinder audiences from supporting the advocacy goal. If audiences do not feel confident about adopting the recommended action presented in messages, they may not become involved (Witte, 1992). In order to circumvent this, message designers need to anticipate and address possible barriers that audiences may face. Barriers may come in two forms—external or internal (Allison, Dwyer, & Makin, 1999).

Internal barriers are constraints and disturbances within the individual that may impede the individual from taking a certain action (Allison et al., 1999). Examples of internal barriers include discomfort, stress, anxiety, uncertainty, fear, misperceptions, among others. To illustrate, audiences may have the misperception that there is a black market for organ donation (Morgan, Harrison, Afifi, Long, & Stephenson, 2008) and therefore disregard advocacy messages calling for signatures to petition for more organ donation facilities. Message designers need to consider such internal barriers and through messaging suggest ways for the audience to overcome those barriers. One possible approach would be to explicitly address the misperceptions audiences have and explain how the misperceptions are erroneous. Message designers also should be mindful not to offend audiences when they point out that the notions audiences hold are inaccurate. Also, people from different cultures may experience different internal barriers. For instance, certain cultural groups may trust doctors less or have less positive attitudes about organ donation (Alden & Cheung, 2000). Message designers may need to cater to different cultural groups accordingly so that these groups may have their internal barriers addressed too. For example, messages targeted toward cultural groups that trust doctors should emphasize the credibility of doctors in order to mitigate the lack of trust.

External barriers are environmental circumstances that may obstruct an individual from taking a certain action. Examples of external barriers include monetary costs, infrastructure problems, distance, lacking access to technology, among others. For instance, if some members of the audience do not have Internet access, an external barrier may be present as they cannot support advocacy efforts that require Internet access, such as in signing an online petition. Message designers need to anticipate such barriers and provide necessary instructions for audiences to circumvent those barriers. For instance, messages targeted toward audiences who lack Internet access and cannot sign an online petition should recommend alternatives such as a physical petition booth. When barriers are addressed in messages, audiences may be more encouraged to participate in advocacy.

Culturally Consistent

Advocacy messages should incorporate cultural elements where appropriate. According to Kreuter and Haughton (2006), when health information integrates culture that is relevant and appropriate for a specific audience, the information captures attention better and helps in stimulating information processing in that audience. One way that messages may incorporate cultural elements is "tailoring" (Hawkins, Kreuter, Resnicow, Fishbein, & Dijkstra, 2008). Tailoring involves the crafting of a message so that the message would specifically attend to the needs and preferences of audiences belonging to a cultural group. Besides tailoring, Kreuter, Lukwago, Bucholtz, Clark, and Sanders-Thompson (2003) recommended five other ways to integrate cultural elements into messages: peripheral, evidential, linguistic, constituent-involving, and socio-cultural approaches.

The peripheral approach relies on aspects that are not within the content of a message (see Petty & Cacioppo, 1984). An example of a peripheral aspect would be color because various cultures identify more or less with certain colors. For instance, Chan and Courtney (2001) found that Hong Kong Chinese strongly associated the color red with danger. In another study, Ou, Luo, Woodcock, and Wright (2004) reported that Chinese participants had a preference for colors that were classified as clean, fresh, or modern. Furthermore, the authors reported that Chinese and British participants associated different colors for the same emotion. In application, message designers should consider the target audiences' preferences for peripheral aspects such as color, type of background music, style of word font, among others. Continuing from the previous example, advocacy messages targeting Hong Kong Chinese could include the color red in order to convey a sense of urgency and danger so that audiences may be motivated to take action and support the advocacy effort. Message designers should conduct a focus group session in order to understand what the preferences for peripheral aspects are for audiences (refer to the section "Pre-Test Draft Advocacy Messages" in Chapter 7 for an explanation on focus groups).

The evidential approach uses information concerning a specific cultural group to address an issue. For example, the evidential approach is used when a message communicates the prevalence of an illness in African Americans to an African American audience. When audiences are given information about people they associate with, they may regard the message as being more relevant and thus take the message more seriously. According to Kreuter and colleagues (2003), the perception that an issue affects similar others may compel audiences to think about the issue, decide to take preventive action, and make plans to act. In application, message designers should find out the most up-to-date information concerning the particular cultural group that the advocacy team is targeting and utilize information where appropriate and relevant. For example, if the advocacy team wants to advocate for better treatment affordability for cancer patients, and there are a significant number of African Americans who have cancer, message designers may want to include the statistical evidence of cancer prevalence among African Americans when communicating the advocacy goal to an African American audience. In this way, the audience may identify more with the problem of expensive cancer treatment and become more motivated to support the advocacy effort.

The linguistic strategy involves using language that is most familiar to a specific cultural group in messages. Message designers may choose to use a specific language with their audiences, such as Spanish for Latin Americans, Mandarin for Asians, French for audiences in France, Bahasa Melayu for audiences in Malaysia, and so on. This approach is not limited to native language, but also includes how a language is spoken within a culture. For instance, African Americans speak English, but there might be nuances in the way they speak English that they better identify with (Squires, 2000). Accordingly, message designers should consider the language target audiences identify most with and how the language is spoken.

The constituent-involving strategy incorporates the experiences of members of a cultural group. For example, a message that shows an African American woman's testimonial about struggling with cancer treatment expenses utilizes the constituent-involving approach. This approach bears resemblance to the evidential approach mentioned previously. Both approaches provide evidence that strengthen the advocacy cause, but the constituent-involving approach differs in that it presents the evidence in a more personal manner by using a representative member of the cultural group to present the evidence. Constituent-involving strategies such as testimonials are effective as they also may draw upon the benefits of using linguistics (Kreuter et al., 2003), disclosure (Han, 2009), and similar others (Kreuter et al., 2003).

Lastly, the socio-cultural approach emphasizes the social structure that a culture is constructed upon. For example, when communicating to a Hispanic audience, a message should reflect core Hispanic values such as "simpatia," which is the need for smooth interpersonal relationships in which confrontation is undesirable (Huerta & Macario, 1999). Therefore, a message such as a video encouraging advocacy participation should be amicable in tone and not threatening in persuading a Hispanic audience to participate in advocacy. Emphasizing the social structure of a culture may make a message more relatable and appealing to audiences belonging to that culture (Kreuter & Haughton, 2006; Kreuter et al., 2003). However, message designers ought to be careful of stereotyping (see e.g., Verhaeghen, Aikman, & Van Gulick, 2011), because audiences may react adversely if they sense that there is stereotyping in messages.

Resource Contingent

The resource capabilities of an advocacy team should be taken into account when developing messages. According to Brady, Verba, and Schlozman (1995), time, money, and communication and organizational skills are resources essential for political participation. Since advocacy involves political participation, these resources pertain to advocacy teams as well. Accordingly, an advocacy team should ascertain how much of these resources are available to them in developing messages.

Time can be important to an advocacy team in three ways. First, an advocacy campaign should not drag on for so long as to become tiresome for the people involved in the campaign, including members of the team and people supporting the advocacy effort. If an advocacy effort is prolonged without bearing fruitful outcomes, team members may become discouraged and restless. This does not mean that campaigns which are lengthy in duration are necessarily problematic; some campaigns naturally require a long time to complete. Rather, this means that campaigns should not be unnecessarily

long; advocacy campaigns should be efficiently carried out. Message designers have to be deliberate, decisive, and on time with message planning and
development. When message designers procrastinate and delay, it can disrupt
progression and result in an unnecessarily lengthy campaign. Supporters of
the campaign may experience fatigue, too, when campaigns drag on for too
long. If an advocacy campaign stirs up excitement in supporters by emphasizing policy changes affecting health, but the advocacy campaign is very slow
in advancing its efforts, supporters may lose the adrenaline they initially had
and may become too exhausted to continue supporting the advocacy effort.
To avoid such a situation, message designers have to be very efficient and
plan ahead. In particular, message designers have to be well-coordinated and
timely with message development.

Second, time is crucial for an advocacy team when there is a deadline to be
met. For example, an advocacy team should disseminate messages before the
legislative session or budget cycle because legislators may be most busy when
the session or cycle begins, and the team wants to avoid its messages being lost
in the busyness (see Gregrich, 2003). In this case, the start of the legislative
session or budget cycle serves as a deadline for the advocacy team. Failure to
meet a deadline may have detrimental consequences for an advocacy team,
and in this instance a team which does not meet the deadline may have to
wait another year or risk delivering messages to preoccupied legislators busy
with the legislative session and budget discussions. Also, an advocacy team
may have self-imposed deadlines to keep the team on track with meeting advocacy goals and be more deliberate with progress toward those goals.

Third, timing can be critical because politicians may not always be available. As mentioned previously, legislators often are most busy when the legislative session or budget cycle begins (see Gregrich, 2003). Therefore an advocacy
team needs to anticipate and prepare ahead and deliver advocacy messages when
legislators are most available. To be sure, legislators can be busy on a regular
basis and not only busy periodically. This is when a lobbyist can be very helpful
for an advocacy team as a lobbyist may negotiate scheduling with legislators so
that the advocacy team can dialogue with relevant legislators.

Time is an important resource that advocacy teams need to manage well
and effectively. When a team wastes time, members of the team and its supporters may experience fatigue. Also, failure to keep track of deadlines may
have detrimental consequences for an advocacy campaign. Politicians oftentimes are busy and therefore timing is crucial as advocacy messages need to
be delivered successfully to legislators without them being preoccupied. An

advocacy team needs to handle time resourcefully in order to avoid the consequences of time mismanagement.

Money is another resource that advocacy teams must take into consideration. An advocacy team may choose to design their own messages or recruit the services of a professional message designer. In the latter case, the advocacy team may have to pay for such services. In the same vein, disseminating advocacy messages through social media can be done by the advocacy team for little to no cost, but disseminating the messages through social media *effectively* may require the skills of a paid professional. In message development, an advocacy team has to determine the aesthetics and reach they want their messages to have and consider if they have the necessary skills to design and deliver the messages they develop. If it is beyond their abilities, then a professional should be enlisted, and money would have to be expended. If a professional message designer is too costly, the advocacy team may choose to raise funds to pay for the expenses, or decide to cut down on the elaborateness of their messages so that a simpler design may incur less costs.

Lastly, the advocacy team should consider the availability of members who are proficient in communication and organizational skills. Such skills include being articulate in discourse, effective in relaying information, and being comfortable in organizing and attending meetings (Brady et al., 1995). These skills are instrumental for advancing messages, and thus the availability of such members should be taken into account in message planning. A person with strong communication and organizational skills may include the communication specialist described in Chapter 3 of this book, or any individual who is confident and competent in adopting the role of a spokesperson and active campaigner for the advocacy team. Such a person should be strong in public speaking and active in delivering advocacy messages to the team's targeted audiences.

Time, money, communication, and organizational skills are important resources to promote political participation and effective advocacy efforts. Accordingly, an advocacy team should address the availability of these resources in message development and work within the ambit of available resources.

Summary

The messaging process in the Health Communication Advocacy Model is crucial to advancing an advocacy effort. By crafting effective advocacy messages, an advocacy team may better capture the attention of target audiences and persuade people to be in favor of the advocacy campaign. There are five key attributes of successful messages: stimulating, motivational, eliminating barriers, culturally consistent, and within the resource capabilities of the organization. When these qualities are integrated into advocacy messages, the messages may be more compelling and effective. Beside these five key elements, message designers also should consider the marketing mix when developing advocacy messages. The marketing mix is elaborated upon in the following chapter.

References

Alden, D. L., & Cheung, A. H. (2000). Organ donation and culture: A comparison of Asian American and European American beliefs, attitudes, and behaviors. *Journal of Applied Social Psychology, 30*(2), 293–314. doi: 10.1111/j.1559–1816.2000.tb02317.x

Allison, K. R., Dwyer, J. J., & Makin, S. (1999). Self-efficacy and participation in vigorous physical activity by high school students. *Health Education & Behavior, 26*(1), 12–24. doi: 10.1177/109019819902600103

Appiah, O. (2006). Rich media, poor media: The impact of audio/video vs. text/picture testimonial ads on browsers' evaluations of commercial web sites and online products. *Journal of Current Issues & Research in Advertising (CTC Press), 28*(1), 73–86. doi: 10.1080/10641734.2006.10505192

Banbury, S. P., Macken, W. J., Tremblay, S., & Jones, D. M., (2001). Auditory distraction and short-term memory: Phenomena and practical implications. *Human Factors: The Journal of the Human Factors and Ergonomics Society, 43*(1), 12–29. doi: 10.1518/001872001775992462

Bradley, M. M., Greenwald, M. K., Petry, M. C., & Lang, P. J. (1992). Remembering pictures: Pleasure and arousal in memory. *Journal of Experimental Psychology: Learning, Memory, and Cognition, 18*(2), 379–390. doi:10.1037/0278–7393.18.2.379

Bradley, M. M., & Lang, P. J. (2000). Affective reactions to acoustic stimuli. *Psychophysiology, 37*(2), 204–215. doi: 10.1111/1469–8986.3720204

Brady, H. E., Verba, S., & Schlozman, K. L. (1995). Beyond SES: A resource model of political participation. *The American Political Science Review, 89*(2), 271–294. Retrieved from http://www.apsanet.org/

Chan, A. H., & Courtney, A. J. (2001). Color associations for Hong Kong Chinese. *International Journal of Industrial Ergonomics, 28*(3), 165–170. doi: 10.1016/S0169–8141(01)00029–4

Collins, N. L., & Miller, L. (1994). Self-disclosure and liking: A meta-analytic review. *Psychological Bulletin, 116*(3), 457–475. doi:10.1037/0033–2909.116.3.457

Coulter, R., Cotte, J., & Moore, M. (1999). Believe it or not: Persuasion, manipulation and credibility of guilt appeals. *Advances in Consumer Research, 26*(1), 288–294. Retrieved from http://www.acrweb.org/

Dubay, L., Holahan, J., & Cook, A. (2007). The uninsured and the affordability of health insurance coverage. *Health Affairs*, 26(1), w22–w30. doi: 10.1377/hlthaff.26.1.w22

Ebbeling, C. B., Pawlak, D. B., & Ludwig, D. S. (2002). Childhood obesity: Public-health crisis, common sense cure. *The Lancet*, 360(9331), 473–482. doi: 10.1016/S0140–6736 (02)09678–2

Gregrich, R. J. (2003). A note to researchers: Communicating science to policy makers and practitioners. *Journal of Substance Abuse Treatment*, 25(3), 233–237. doi: 10.1016/S0740–5472(03)00120-X

Guttman, N., & Salmon, C. T. (2004). Guilt, fear, stigma and knowledge gaps: Ethical issues in public health communication interventions. *Bioethics*, 18(6), 531–552. doi:10.1111/j.1467–8519.2004.00415.x

Han, H. C. (2009). Does the content of political appeals matter in motivating participation? A field experiment on self-disclosure in political appeals. *Political Behavior*, 31(1), 103–116. doi: 10.1007/s11109–008–9066–9

Hawkins, R. P., Kreuter, M., Resnicow, K., Fishbein, M., & Dijkstra, A. (2008). Understanding tailoring in communicating about health. *Health Education Research*, 23(3), 454–466. doi: 10.1093/her/cyn004

Huerta, E. E., & Macario, E. (1999). Communicating health risk to ethnic groups: Reaching Hispanics as a case study. *Journal of the National Cancer Institute Monographs*, 1999(25), 23–26. Retrieved from http://jncimono.oxfordjournals.org/

Kreuter, M. W., & Haughton, L. T. (2006). Integrating culture into health information for African American women. *American Behavioral Scientist*, 49(6), 794–811. doi: 10.1177/0002764205283801

Kreuter, M. W., Lukwago, S. N., Bucholtz, D. C., Clark, E. M., & Sanders-Thompson, V. (2003). Achieving cultural appropriateness in health promotion programs: Targeted and tailored approaches. *Health Education & Behavior*, 30(2), 133–146. doi: 10.1177/1090198102251021

Kugler, K., & Jones, W. H. (1992). On conceptualizing and assessing guilt. *Journal of Personality and Social Psychology*, 62(2), 318–327. doi:10.1037/0022–3514.62.2.318

Lang, A., Dhillon, K., & Dong, Q. (1995). The effects of emotional arousal and valence on television viewers' cognitive capacity and memory. *Journal of Broadcasting & Electronic Media*, 39(3), 313–327. doi: 10.1080/08838159509364309

Mattson, M. (2010). Health advocacy by accident and discipline. *Health Communication*, 25(6–7), 622–624. doi: 10.1080/10410236.2010.496844

Moore, D. J., Harris, W. D., & Chen, H. C. (1995). Affect intensity: An individual difference response to advertising appeals. *Journal of Consumer Research*, 22(2), 154–164. Retrieved from http://www.journals.uchicago.edu/

Morgan, S. E., Harrison, T. R., Afifi, W. A., Long, S. D., & Stephenson, M. T. (2008). In their own words: The reasons why people will (not) sign an organ donor card. *Health Communication*, 23(1), 23–33. doi: 10.1080/10410230701805158

Nabi, R. L. (1999). A cognitive-functional model for the effects of discrete negative emotions on information processing, attitude change, and recall. *Communication Theory*, 9(3), 292–320. doi: 10.1111/j.1468–2885.1999.tb00172.x

O'Keefe, D. J. (2002). Guilt as a mechanism of persuasion. In J. P. Dillard & M. Pfau (Eds.), *The persuasion handbook: Developments in theory and practice* (pp. 329–344). Thousand Oaks, CA: Sage.

Ou, L. C., Luo, M. R., Woodcock, A., & Wright, A. (2004). A study of colour emotion and colour preference. Part I: Colour emotions for single colours. *Color Research & Application*, 29(3), 232–240. doi: 10.1002/col.20010

Petty, R. E., & Cacioppo, J. T. (1984). The effects of involvement on responses to argument quantity and quality: Central and peripheral routes to persuasion. *Journal of Personality and Social Psychology*, 46(1), 69–81. doi:10.1037/0022–3514.46.1.69

Potter, R. F. (2000). The effects of voice changes on orienting and immediate cognitive overload in radio listeners. *Media Psychology*, 2(2), 147–177. doi: 10.1207/S1532785XMEP0202_3

Randolph, W., & Viswanath, K. K. (2004). Lessons learned from public health mass media campaigns: Marketing health in a crowded media world. *Annual Review of Public Health*, 25(1), 419–437. doi:10.1146/annurev.publhealth.25.101802.123046

Ravaja, N. (2004). Effects of image motion on a small screen on emotion, attention, and memory: Moving-face versus static-face newscaster. *Journal of Broadcasting & Electronic Media*, 48(1), 108–133. Retrieved from http://www.tandf.co.uk/journals/HBEM

Rodero, E. (2012). See it on a radio story sound effects and shots to evoked imagery and attention on audio fiction. *Communication Research*, 39(4), 458–479. doi: 10.1177/0093650210386947

Ruiter, R. C., Abraham, C., & Kok, G. (2001). Scary warnings and rational precautions: A review of the psychology of fear appeals. *Psychology & Health*, 16(6), 613–630. Retrieved from http://www.tandf.co.uk/journals/titles/08870446.asp

Smith, S. M., & Shaffer, D. R. (2000). Vividness can undermine or enhance message processing: The moderating role of vividness congruency. *Personality and Social Psychology Bulletin*, 26(7), 769–779. doi: 10.1177/0146167200269003

Squires, C. R. (2000). Black talk radio: Defining community needs and identity. *The Harvard International Journal of Press/Politics*, 5(2), 73–95.

Swinburn, B. A., Sacks, G., Hall, K. D., McPherson, K., Finegood, D. T., Moodie, M. L., & Gortmaker, S. L. (2011). The global obesity pandemic: Shaped by global drivers and local environments. *The Lancet*, 378(9793), 804–814. doi: 10.1016/S0140–6736(11)60813–1

Turner, M. M. (2007). Using emotion in risk communication: The anger activism model. *Public Relations Review*, 33(2), 114–119. doi: 10.1016/j.pubrev.2006.11.013

Turner, M. M. (2012). Using emotional appeals in health messages. In Hyunyi Cho (Ed.), *Health communication message design: theory and practice* (pp. 59–71). Thousand Oaks, CA: Sage.

Venkatraman, M. P., Marlino, D., Kardes, F. R., & Sklar, K. B. (1990). The interactive effects of message appeal and individual differences on information processing and persuasion. *Psychology & Marketing*, 7(2), 85–96. doi: 10.1002/mar.4220070202

Verhaeghen, P., Aikman, S. N., & Van Gulick, A. E. (2011). Prime and prejudice: Co-occurrence in the culture as a source of automatic stereotype priming. *British Journal of Social Psychology*, 50(3), 501–518. doi:10.1348/014466610X524254

Witte, K. (1991). *Preventing AIDS through persuasive communications: Fear appeals and preventive-action efficacy.* Unpublished doctoral dissertation, University of California, Irvine.

Witte, K. (1992). Putting the fear back into fear appeals: The extended parallel process model. *Communications Monographs, 59*(4), 329–349. doi: 10.1080/03637759209376276

Witte, K. (1994). Fear control and danger control: A test of the extended parallel process model (EPPM). *Communications Monographs, 61*(2), 113–134. doi: 10.1080/03637759409376328

Witte, K., & Allen, M. (2000). A meta-analysis of fear appeals: Implications for effective public health campaigns. *Health Education & Behavior, 27*(5), 591–615. doi: 10.1177/109019810002700506

· 7 ·

MARKETING MIX

In 1971, Kotler and Zaltman ushered in a new wave of campaign research and practice when they introduced the concept of social marketing. Previously, marketing mostly was thought about in the context of businesses selling goods to consumers. Kotler and Zaltman's concept of social marketing changed this perspective as the authors applied marketing strategies for the purposes of generating social action. Thus, instead of persuading consumers to purchase goods, social marketing involves persuading people to take social action, such as donating to charities, engaging in healthier lifestyles, or supporting an advocacy effort.

The marketing mix is a term which describes the aspects of social marketing which are most important for achieving a successful social marketing endeavor, and sometimes it is referred to as the four Ps. The marketing mix is composed of product, price, placement, and promotion. Because social marketing is about persuading people to take social action, the importance of incorporating the marketing mix into advocacy messages is essential. In this chapter, each element of the marketing mix will be defined and examples will be presented accordingly.

Product

Product in the marketing mix refers to the recommended social action and how it is presented to target audiences. In the context of health advocacy, the product would be the notion of supporting the advocacy effort. For example, an advocacy team may have "support prosthetic parity" as its product. One may imagine the banners that often appear in advocacy campaigns as the advertisements for the advocacy product. In other words, these banners often-times describe the product of an advocacy team. If a banner exclaims "Support us for better cancer treatment affordability!," then the product is exactly what the banner says. Also, the positional statement described in Chapter 3 usually hints to what the product is. For example, if an advocacy team's positional statement is "to pass legislation to provide more facilities for the blind in parks," then the likely product presented to target audiences would be "to support the call for more facilities for the blind in parks." Like businesses that persuade consumers to buy their products, the aim of advocacy teams is to per-suade people to "buy" their product. That is, to support the advocacy effort.

Like tangible products that businesses sell, advocacy teams need to know how to "brand" their call for action and how to make it persuasive and ap-pealing to target audiences. In order to achieve this, advocacy teams first have to understand the needs of their target audiences (Kotler & Zaltman, 1971). For instance, if an advocacy team is targeting youths, what themes would be most relevant for youths? What themes would be most appealing for them? To illustrate, adolescents may be high sensation-seeking and thus messages that induce high sensation may address them better; conversely, low sensa-tion messages would not appeal to these adolescents (Stephenson, 2003). Thus, message designers may want to craft messages such that the messages may be exciting to the youthful audience. Message designers may achieve this by including more stimulating elements in messages as described previously in Chapter 6, such as loud noises, catchy rhythms, tense music, fast-moving visuals, and emotionally arousing scenes, among others. The preferences of audiences may be very subtle, such as the preferences for certain font type-faces (see Buehner, 2011). Continuing with the example of youths as the tar-get audience, do the youths prefer classic, cursive, or trendier font typefaces? Do they prefer striking colors for words used in a poster, or are multi-colored words more appealing to them? Message designers need a good eye for de-tail to determine what appeals most to target audiences. A good approach to ascertain the preferences of a target audience is conducting pre-testing of draft advocacy messages. Pre-testing allows message designers to determine even the more subtle preferences that audiences may have such as color and typeface (pre-testing will be described at greater length toward the end of this chapter). Besides aesthetic appeals, an advocacy team also would have to consider how to make the content appealing to audiences. In the example of youths as a target audience, crafting the content of an advocacy message such that it would be appealing to youths can be a difficult task, as youths may be less interested in political participation (Quintelier, 2007). In such cases, advocacy teams need to obtain feedback from youths to understand what the pertinent issues are for youths. After getting the feedback, message designers should frame the content of the advocacy messages based on the feedback so that it would relate to youths. When attention is given to the aesthetic and content appeals of the advocacy product, target audiences may be more compelled to consider the product and support the advocacy effort.

Price

In social marketing, price refers to the cost incurred by the audience to engage in the social action, and includes psychological, monetary, energy, or opportunity costs (Kotler & Zaltman, 1971). Advocacy message designers should take into account the burdens that audiences may potentially experience in carrying out the recommended action of the advocacy message. Message designers can address concerns about potential costs to mitigate audiences' fears associated with the various types of costs.

Psychological costs are internal constraints and disturbances within an individual and are similar to the internal barriers described previously in Chapter 6. Psychological costs may include discomfort, stress, anxiety, uncertainty, and fear, among others. For example, there may be people who feel uncertain about signing a petition. They may be apprehensive because of a belief that there may be negative consequences in supporting an advocacy effort. Some individuals may fear that their signature may be used for a purpose other than the advocated health issue. Some also may feel hesitant to sign a petition because they do not know what level of involvement they may have to commit to after signing a petition. For instance, they may have the impression that they could be liable for court or legal matters. Also, some people may be concerned that, after signing a petition, an advocacy team might keep harassing them for future support, and use their signature as a pressuring reminder of their commitment to the cause. Of course, a legitimate health advocacy team would not function in these inappropriate ways and signing a petition should not pull an individual into complicated legal or court issues. However, there may be people who still hold such perceptions, and message designers may need to consider how to assuage these potential fears in some audience members. One approach an advocacy team may adopt is to briefly discuss with audiences at a petition booth that people who sign the petition are safe from legal complications and that their involvement is limited to supporting that single campaign through petitioning. By briefly discussing with audiences such potential concerns, those who were worried about such matters may become more confident and assured and thus support the campaign through petition. Furthermore, audiences who were not concerned about such issues may be more persuaded to support the advocacy effort as the advocacy team may show itself to be a reliable and thoughtful team by addressing those concerns.

Another common advocacy method that may draw concerns in audiences is rallying. To rally is to convene with a group of people to raise awareness about a certain issue. Rallying may be of concern to potential supporters because of the uncertainty it can bring. For example, one may be worried about being unable to remain anonymous. Although the very nature of rallying does not enable anonymity, an advocacy team can try to persuade potential supporters that the goal is laudable, and if the crowd is large enough personal identification may not be a concern; in fact, one may even desire his or her participation to be made known since the goal is laudable. Also, potential supporters may experience anxiety if they are uncertain about the proceedings of the rally, such as where exactly to convene, what their expected role in rallying is, or what the expected outcome of the rally is. These uncertainties can be circumvented by briefing those who may participate about what is expected during the rally. Accordingly, an advocacy team should inform rallying participants of the exact location and time for assembly, and the site should be a landmark which is easy to find and accessible.

An important topic to discuss during the briefing is the role of the rallying participants. The roles of participants must be made clear so that participants feel prepared and confident for the rally. For instance, an advocacy team may brief participants that their role is to gather together and hold signs that promote awareness about a health issue. In such a scenario, the advocacy team should not assume that participants would design their own banners and signboards and would bring these items along to the rally. Instead, an advocacy team should take the initiative and supply for participants any necessary items for the rally, which may include designing and creating the signs. An advocacy team also should explain to rallying participants what the purpose and expected outcome of the rally is. Because rallying is a concerted effort, a rally that has individuals with their own agendas may compromise the harmony and goal of the rallying group. For example, if some individuals believe that the rallying outcome is to present the advocacy cause to legislators, but others in the rallying group think the purpose of the rally is to present the advocacy cause to a news reporting crew, then there may be confusion and fractions within the rallying group, and such disharmony in the group may jeopardize the rallying effort. Therefore, an advocacy team should prevent such uncertainty in supporters by explaining the rallying purpose and expected outcome. For instance, an advocacy team may say to supporters prior to the rally that the purpose of the rally is to present the advocacy cause to a news reporting crew and the expected outcome is that the advocacy message would be further spread through the news report. In that manner, an advocacy team can prevent psychological costs such as anxiety, uncertainty, and confusion. In turn, audiences who listen to the explanation of the advocacy team would view the costs of participation as being lesser and may consequently become more persuaded to participate.

Another potential cost that audiences may incur in supporting an advocacy effort is monetary cost. For instance, an advocacy team may have a fundraising campaign to cover expenses, such as in hiring a lobbyist. In such a scenario, the product of the advocacy message may be to support the advocacy goal through donation. The price, then, would be the amount which an audience gives for donation. It is important for an advocacy team to be transparent and clear in how they are using the funds raised, so that audiences may feel assured and be persuaded to donate, and donors may not feel uneasy about how the money is spent. Apart from raising funds, there rarely are significant monetary costs for audiences of a health advocacy campaign. There often is little monetary cost for supporting an advocacy goal through signing a petition, attending a rally, among other advocacy activities. However, when target audiences are legislators, monetary costs can become a more significant concern. For example, when an advocacy team tries to persuade legislation to allocate more of a state's resources into building more facilities for cancer treatment, the monetary considerations are essential. In such situations, an advocacy team should have an estimate of how much the expenses would be.

This estimate should have been accounted for during the formative research phase previously described in Chapter 5. An advocacy team can ask related experts such as hospital developers or executives who manage hospitals for an estimate of such expenses. It also would be helpful for the advocacy team to have already enlisted such an expert to be a member of the team during the assembling of the advocacy team discussed previously in Chapter 3. Alternatively, if the advocacy team cannot contact such an expert, the team should try researching on the Internet for information. An advocacy team would not appear very convincing if it does not know the cost of its own product. Therefore, a team should obtain the best possible approximation so that they may appear informed and the legislators may be more effectively persuaded.

Energy cost is the physical effort required of audiences to support an advocacy goal. Similar to psychological cost, an important concern that audiences may have is the level of commitment they need to support the advocacy goal. For example, if a rally is stipulated to happen during the morning in a location far away from residences, audiences may not be compelled to participate as the physical effort required in waking up early and travelling far away might make the notion of participation too unattractive to merit participation (see also Gimpel & Schuknecht, 2003). Therefore, an advocacy team should try to reduce energy costs as much as possible so that advocacy messages may be more appealing. For example, instead of suggesting a morning rally far away from residences, an advocacy team may be able to persuade audiences to participate in an evening rally in a close-by town. Alternatively, the advocacy team could suggest to audiences that they may support the advocacy campaign by signing an online petition that could be referred to at a rally. Energy cost also is important when the audience is the media. If an advocacy team wants to persuade media to broadcast news about its advocacy campaign, but the rally is conducted in a faraway location, the energy costs required of the news crew to travel such a distance may dissuade the media from providing news coverage of the advocacy campaign. Therefore, an advocacy team should seek to minimize energy costs and communicate that the physical effort required to support the advocacy goal is minimal.

Opportunity cost is the sacrifice of alternatives due to a decision made (Burch & Henry, 1974). For example, an individual may have to forgo a relaxing weekend at the swimming pool based on a decision to attend a rally during the weekend. Although opportunity cost may not be immediately apparent to an advocacy team, a little thoughtful consideration may enable the team to estimate what the opportunity cost may be for audiences. For instance, if the targeted audience is middle-class working adults, an advocacy team should probably assume that weekends are valuable for this audience as weekends are for relaxation, leisure, and family time. Thus, if an advocacy team schedules a rally for the weekend, there likely is a great opportunity cost for a member of that audience to participate in a rally. A participant may have to sacrifice a fun time at the beach or a picnic with the family in order to attend the rally. In such a scenario, an advocacy team should not expect much attendance for the rally. Instead, a rally may be better attended if scheduled on a weekday such as Friday. Since adult audiences often are working, their opportunity cost usually involves the compromise of leisure time. Because leisure time may be highly valued among working adults, an advocacy team will want to consider platforms for these audiences to support that are not too time-consuming. For instance, signing petitions online would not involve much time. Accordingly, an advocacy team should ascertain the preferences of audiences and the manner in which audiences may spend their time, and then schedule advocacy events that involve the least opportunity cost for audiences.

Another way that advocacy teams could address opportunity costs is to communicate to audiences that the sacrifice is worth it. In some instances, the opportunity cost almost always is very large. Especially with working adults, some may feel that supporting an advocacy campaign may be a costly effort involving loss of wages or leisure time with little or no personally beneficial returns. Although supporting a health advocacy campaign may not personally benefit such audiences, an advocacy team should emphasize to these audiences that their support can help the lives of many others. Thus, an advocacy team should explain to such audiences that their sacrifices are justified and worth the costs. The team may communicate this to audiences using the emotionally stimulating and motivational techniques for messages described previously in Chapter 6.

When the target audience is the media, their opportunity cost may be the news coverage they could have had if not for their coverage on the advocacy team's campaign. In this case, the advocacy team should design messages that would persuade the media that the advocacy campaign is newsworthy. Because media often have sensationalistic approaches to covering news (see e.g., Caulfield & Bubela, 2004; Grabe, Zhou, & Barnett, 2001), an advocacy team has to convince the media that the advocacy campaign has engaging elements suitable for news coverage. An advocacy team can persuade the media by communicating to the media their advocacy campaign in a stimulating way, which is an approach that was discussed previously in Chapter 6. For example, an advocacy team campaigning for prosthetic parity may inform the media that a large group of amputees will be rallying with banners and signboards outside a statehouse on a particular day. The rally would likely attract much attention, and thus the media may likely be persuaded to give news coverage on the advocacy campaign and its rally. In general, whoever the audience may be, an advocacy team should convince the audience that their support of the advocacy campaign is worth investing in as compared to the alternatives forgone.

Every product has a price, and in social marketing, price often includes psychological, monetary, energy, and opportunity costs. In health advocacy, these costs are pertinent to audiences who wish to support an advocacy goal. An advocacy team has to consider the relevant costs and mitigate those costs as much as possible. Advocacy messages should address those costs and convince audiences that the costs are minimal or that supporting the advocacy campaign is worth the costs involved.

Place

In social marketing, place refers to the channel for audiences to translate motivation into action (Kotler & Zaltman, 1971). It is through a channel that audiences are able to support the advocacy goal, and it is the responsibility of an advocacy team to direct audiences to an appropriate channel. The channel can be a physical location, such as a petition booth or rally site, or it could be nonphysical, such as the Internet (e.g., online petition, social media) or traditional media (e.g., radio, television news, newspapers). In this section, each of these channels will be elaborated upon respectively.

A physical location such as a petition booth is a common channel for advocacy. A petition booth is an excellent channel because it does not involve complicated procedures; audiences simply have to go to the booth and sign the petition. Also, signing a petition does not require much input from an audience member; audiences do not have to contribute financially or be actively involved in the campaign. Rather, audiences sign a petition to show that they are in favor of an advocacy goal and do not need further involvement. Thus, a petition booth is an effective channel because signing a petition is convenient for audiences and does not demand much from them. An advocacy team should set up a petition booth in a location where many people frequent because a popular site can help promote awareness for the advocacy campaign and allow supporters to locate the booth easily. An advocacy team also should decorate the petition booth with banners and make it stand out with bright colors such as yellow or red to draw attention. The more petition signatures an advocacy team has, the more persuasive the team can be when communicating to legislators. This is because the advocated health issue is no longer just the concern of the advocacy team, but the signatures show that the health concern pertains to hundreds (and possibly thousands) of other state members as well, all of whom state legislators are supposed to serve.

The downsides of having a physical location for a channel are its susceptibility to bad weather and that audiences may deem the location too far away for them. Bad weather such as rain may render a petition booth inaccessible, and the channel would not be an effective one in such circumstances as there likely would not be much turnout. Instead a petition booth can be set up inside a building such as a shopping mall, but doing so requires the permission of the building management, which can be a complicated and onerous process. Even if permission is granted, audience turnout may still be low as people may choose to stay at home because of the rain. When there is good weather, some individuals still may not visit the petition booth because they may deem it too far away for them. For such individuals, it may be best to direct them to alternative channels such as a nonphysical online petition.

Another physical location that can be an advocacy channel is a rallying site. By participating in a rally, participants show their overt support for an advocacy campaign. Conducting a rally can be advantageous for an advocacy team because it can promote a lot of awareness; participants oftentimes are excited and highly motivated during a rally and such an energetic crowd usually draws much attention. As aforementioned, conducting a rally requires planning and briefing. An advocacy team must plan beforehand which location would be most appropriate to advance the advocacy goal through rallying. For instance, conducting a rally in a popular area in a city can draw a lot of attention if the advocacy team feels that promoting awareness is needed for reaching the advocacy goal. Alternatively, the rally can be conducted outside a statehouse if the advocacy team feels that doing so would help draw the attention of legislators and compel them to dialogue with the advocacy team. If an advocacy team feels that dialogue with legislators is necessary to reach the advocacy goal, then conducting the rally outside a statehouse may be a strategic option. Planning is crucial for a rally because the advocacy team needs to inform participants what needs to be done to accomplish the goals of the rally.

Although participants may be enthusiastic and excited to take part in a rally, excitement cannot take the place of preparedness. For example, an advocacy team must not assume that participants will create and bring signs or banners to the rally. Instead, the team should design and supply signs and banners for participants to carry during the rally. The advocacy team also should clearly inform participants that signs and banners provided by the advocacy team are preferred for the rally. This is important as it helps to avoid conflicting or incongruent messages. As previously mentioned, bad weather conditions may compromise channels that use physical locations, so an advocacy team has to consider a contingency plan for such situations. For instance, the rally can be postponed to another day. However, doing so may dampen the motivation and excitement of the participants. This is a downside to physical channels that an advocacy team has to prepare for; although physical channels often can be very effective for advocacy, such channels can be easily compromised by weather.

Briefing is another important requirement for conducting a rally. Participants often need clear directions from an advocacy team on what needs to be done. In particular, briefing about the role of participants should be provided. Assigning roles to participants can be a tricky task as participants may have preferences about what they want to do. For example, if the rally requires a few participants to be vocal and to chant the words of a banner loudly, and a participant who is timid and prefers a less prominent role is assigned this vocal role, this participant is likely to perform the assigned role less effectively. Furthermore, the participant may become unhappy about the predicament of being assigned such a role, and this unhappiness may become contagious and affect the moods of other participants. If a single misplaced assignment can affect the moods of a few participants, many inappropriate assignments may be very detrimental to the mood of the entire rally. Accordingly, an advocacy team should brief the participants about their roles and ask them during the briefing if anyone would prefer another role. For example, some may find carrying a sign too laborious and prefer handing out pamphlets instead. Or, some participants may have their own cliques and prefer the same roles as their friends. In such cases, assigning the role of holding banners or signs may be a suitable option. As previously mentioned in this chapter, briefing about expected outcomes also is important because it prevents confusion and gives participants a clear sense of direction that they can strive toward. For example, if the purpose of the rally is to promote awareness for the advocated health issue, the expected outcome should be the increase in the number of people who know about the issue. If this expected outcome is made explicit to participants beforehand, participants likely will have a greater sense of confidence and may work toward that outcome collectively. With adequate planning and briefing, a rallying site can be an effective channel for audiences to support an advocacy campaign.

Besides physical locations, nonphysical spaces such as the Internet or more traditional media such as radio and television news also can be effective places for audiences to support an advocacy campaign. There are primarily two ways that the Internet can be used as a place for supporting advocacy. First, audiences may use the Internet to sign online petitions. Second, audiences may show their support of the advocacy campaign through social media such as Facebook.

An online petition is a statement published on the Internet which people can read and sign electronically to show their support (Earl, 2006). According to Earl (2006), online petition providers such as MoveOn.org and PetitionOnline.com have received thousands of signatures for a variety of causes, including petitions against political issues and war. Other social movement organizations, such as the National Organization for Women, also employ online petitions. The use of online petitions also can be extended to advocating for health issues (see e.g., Mattson, 2010). Online petitioning can be an effective channel for advocacy purposes, especially when the number of signatures is very large. Although there is no fixed number for signatures, petitions often include thousands of signatures (see e.g., Earl, 2006; Mattson, 2010). For instance, an online petition against the impeachment of Bill Clinton in 1998 had 500,000 signatures (Earl, 2006). Although 500,000 signatures may not be expected for a health advocacy campaign, such a figure illustrates how potentially compelling online petitioning can be. For health advocacy campaigns, approximately a thousand signatures usually warrants the attention of policymakers (see e.g., Mattson, 2010). Personally designing and hosting an online petition site can be a challenging and laborious task. Therefore, a better approach would be for an advocacy team to use the services of an existing online petition provider such as the aforementioned PetitionOnline.com. Through this channel, audiences are able to show their support for a health advocacy campaign with little to no physical effort. Furthermore, an online petition is a convenient channel that does not require too much of the audience's time and attention. However, not every member of the audience may prefer using an online petition to show their support for an advocacy effort. For example, Xie and Jaeger (2008) reported that older adults are hesitant to engage in political participation via the Internet. Accordingly, an advocacy team must understand who their target audiences are and direct these audiences to the most appropriate channel for supporting the advocacy effort.

Another place that audiences can go to show their support for an advocacy campaign is social media. According to Kaplan and Haenlein (2010), social media is a group of Internet-based applications that users participate in by generating and exchanging web content. Many Internet applications fall under the broad definition of social media, but for the purposes of health advocacy, we consider the use of Facebook in particular. Facebook is a social networking site that began as a college networking site in 2004 and expanded into a site with a global reach (boyd & Ellison, 2007). Facebook can be used as a place for audiences to show their support for a health advocacy campaign. Audiences can show their support by "liking" the advocacy team's group page. In this context, the "liking" function represents being in favor of the team's advocacy cause. Getting many "likes" is akin to getting many signatures for a petition—the greater the number, the more compelling the advocacy can be. There is, however, a caveat. The "likes" on Facebook may not have the sort of persuasive impact that signatures on petitions have when it comes to health advocacy. At best, the number of "likes" can be seen as a supporting argument when dialoguing with policymakers that there are people in favor of the advocacy goal. Furthermore, there is growing literature that suggests a large number of "likes" for an activism-related group page does not necessarily mean strong actual support. For instance, according to Morozov (2012), a popular Facebook cause, Saving the Children of Africa, had over 1.7 million members, but only raised about $12,000. This lack of transition to actual participation is known as "slacktivism," which refers to the willingness to perform a token display of support for a social cause accompanied by a lack of willingness to invest significant effort for meaningful change (Kristofferson, White, & Peloza, 2014). Slacktivism is such a prevalent phenomenon that UNICEF Sweden launched a "Likes Don't Save Lives" campaign to remind people that financial contributions, and not token displays of support, are necessary for helping children in developing nations combat disease (Kristofferson et al., 2014). For a health advocacy campaign, slacktivism may occur when supporters "like" the advocacy team's Facebook page, but do little to contribute to the advocacy effort thereafter, such as not contributing financially during fundraising, not participating in a rally, not signing an online petition, and so on. In regards to signing online petitions, Panagiotopoulos, Sams, Elliman, and Fitzgerald (2011) found that there is little connection between Facebook support and online petition signatures. These researchers discovered many instances where there was high Facebook support which translated into few signatures and also cases where there were many signatures, but Facebook support was limited. Because motivation may not translate into action in social media such as Facebook, and because having support on Facebook may not be very helpful for an advocacy campaign, an advocacy team should use this channel sparingly and with discretion. An advocacy team can use social media such as Facebook as a channel for its audiences, but the team should anticipate and prepare for the minimal beneficial outcomes that are likely when taking such a route. The use of social media such as Facebook for health advocacy is perhaps more advantageous for promotional purposes, which are described later in this chapter.

Besides the Internet, traditional media are another nonphysical channel that audiences can use to show their support for an advocacy cause. The traditional media we consider are radio, television news, and newspapers. Not every audience member can use such channels. For instance, a patient who wants to support a health advocacy campaign cannot simply walk into a news reporting studio and speak favorably about the campaign without permission. Therefore, the media—which are one of the advocacy's audiences described previously in Chapter 5—should be the ones to use such channels as they have access to such avenues. The media can show their support for an advocacy campaign by speaking in favor of it through the radio, television news, or newspapers.

The use of radio as a channel can be effective because it may have considerable reach. Although the radio has been facing competition from more advanced media platforms such as the Internet and podcast (see Albarran et al., 2007), there still are many people who listen to the radio. For instance, many people listen to the radio when they drive a car or truck (Dibben & Williamson, 2007). The media can support a health advocacy campaign by speaking favorably about the campaign on the radio. For example, if an advocacy team had communicated to a radio broadcast station about its advocacy campaign, and the station was persuaded by the advocacy messages, the station could decide to inform its listeners about the campaign and give favorable opinions about it. Also, the radio station may be persuaded to support the health advocacy effort by providing the advocacy team some air time to promote the advocacy cause. Granting access to radio air time through a public service announcement is a valuable form of support as it can be difficult and costly to have a spot on the radio for promoting a health advocacy campaign. A public service announcement is the dedicated time on a media outlet (such as the radio) for addressing social concerns (such as advocated health issues). An advocacy team can benefit greatly from a public service announcement because messages communicated in this manner usually reach many audiences.

Television news and newspapers also are channels that media can utilize to help support an advocacy campaign. Like the radio, television news and newspapers also have been facing competition from more advanced platforms such as online news and satire news, such as *The Daily Show with Jon Stewart* (see Baym, 2005). However, there still are people who watch television news and read newspapers, thus these channels can be useful avenues for supporting advocacy. When an advocacy team successfully persuades a news company with its advocacy messages, the news company may offer to provide news coverage for the advocacy campaign on television or in a newspaper. As an example, Professor Mattson and her advocacy team were conducting a rally outside a statehouse during their campaign for prosthetic parity, and among their audiences was a local news crew which was reporting on something else at that time. The rally and its advocacy message drew the attention of the news crew, and eventually they asked Professor Mattson and her advocacy team if they could report about the advocacy team and the prosthetic parity campaign. Professor Mattson and her advocacy team agreed, and the prosthetic parity campaign was reported in the news at no cost to the advocacy team but with great benefit for the advocacy effort which eventually succeeded.

There are physical and nonphysical places that audiences can go to give support to an advocacy effort, and it is the responsibility of an advocacy team to direct audiences to appropriate channels. Physical locations may include petition booths and rally sites. Nonphysical places include the Internet (e.g., online petition, social media) and traditional media (e.g., radio, television news, newspapers). An advocacy team must ascertain through formative research which placement is most beneficial for the advocacy effort and most appropriate for its audiences, and then recommend that channel to its audiences.

Promotion

Promotion in the marketing mix refers to the act of bringing the product to the attention of audiences (Kotler & Zaltman, 1971). In the context of health advocacy, this means raising awareness about the advocacy effort. Promotion is important because the success of a health advocacy effort is largely dependent on the support of many people. There are many ways in which an advocacy team may promote their campaign, including conducting a rally, using social media, or using traditional media.

A rally is effective for promotional purposes because an enthusiastic crowd holding signboards and banners often piques the curiosity of onlookers. The media also may become curious and report about the rally. An advocacy team should consider informing the media about the rally prior to conducting the rally. In that way, the media will be alerted to this gathering and the likelihood of one or more media outlets reporting on the rally may increase. An advocacy team may choose to distribute pamphlets that provide more information regarding the health advocacy effort during the rally. The pamphlet should contain details such as ways to support the campaign and the advocacy team's contact information. As previously discussed, a rally is susceptible to bad weather and thus using this approach involves the risk of needing to cancel the rally due to bad weather. An advocacy team must anticipate and prepare for such predicaments and plan for alternatives.

Another approach to promote an advocacy effort is to use social media. An advocacy team may promote their cause by using social media such as Facebook and Twitter. Both channels are useful for promotion because both have large number of users. For instance, Facebook had 1 billion active monthly active users at the end of 2012 (Caers et al., 2013) and Twitter has had over 200 million users (Junco, Elavsky, & Heiberger, 2013). Therefore, although there are other social media platforms, Facebook and Twitter are highly recommended because of the popularity of these two channels. Also, other social media platforms may not be well-suited for advocacy purposes. For example, Merry (2010) found that few environmental organizations use blogs and that there is very little interaction between blog authors and readers. For these reasons, Facebook and Twitter are further explored and recommended for health advocacy promotion.

There are several advantages in using Facebook for promoting a health advocacy effort. First, the team can set up a group profile page dedicated to the advocacy campaign and post related information, such as the email and contact details of the advocacy team. Second, a group profile page on Facebook enables the advocacy team to post updates regarding the advocacy effort for its audiences to read. Third, an advocacy team can post videos on Facebook for the advocacy supporters to view. Because of these features that aid promotion, Facebook can be an effective tool for an advocacy team in raising awareness of its campaign. In contrast, Twitter does not have such expansive features, particularly since it has a character limit for writing text messages since it has a character limit for writing text messages. However, recent expansion of the Twitter text limit should provide sufficient space for an advocacy team to post information regarding its campaign. An advocacy team may choose to use both Facebook and Twitter instead of limiting itself to only one social media platform. However, an advocacy team has to first consider whether using two platforms is more beneficial than using only one platform. Also, the team should take into account available campaign resources and consider if the team could use two social media platforms effectively and within resource capabilities.

It should be emphasized that an advocacy team would be facing a lot of competition for audiences' attention if the advocacy team chooses to use social media for promotion; there are many other messages that would be vying for audiences' attention, too, including messages from businesses, activist organizations, and societies, among others. Thus, an advocacy team must utilize the message crafting strategies discussed in Chapter 6 in order to stand out from other messages and gain the attention of target audiences. Another important consideration of an advocacy team is the description of place within promotion. Oftentimes, message designers can become too immersed in the promotional aspect of messaging and forget to sufficiently mention the place where audiences can go to support the advocacy effort.

Traditional media are another approach to promote a health advocacy effort. An advocacy team can advertise through radio or television programs to promote their advocacy effort. However, radio and television advertising can be costly. An advocacy team must determine if there are sufficient financial resources to advertise on radio or television. Even if there are adequate financial resources, it may not be very cost-effective to promote a campaign through radio and television advertising (see Farrelly, Hussin, & Bauer, 2007). In other words, the number of people who become aware of the advocacy campaign may not justify the high costs involved in such advertising. A better approach may be to persuade the media to promote the advocacy effort for no cost, which is known as earned media. Although this may not seem feasible, it actually is very possible to achieve. Because many media outlets often depend on sensationalism (see Grabe et al., 2001), an advocacy effort can be very attractive news for the media, especially when the advocacy effort includes a rally that has people holding signboards and banners. An advocacy team needs to frame the advocacy effort in an attractive way for the media, portraying the campaign such that it seems highly newsworthy and would catch the attention of the media's audiences. Granted, some advocacy campaigns or advocated health issues may not be exciting or newsworthy in nature, but the key to having the media promote the advocacy effort is not how newsworthy the campaign is, but that the campaign *appears* newsworthy. To do that, an advocacy team should utilize the messaging strategies described in Chapter 6. Also, as mentioned previously, a rally can be very enticing for the media because a crowd holding signboards and banners fits the sensationalistic approach that many media outlets use. Thus, the goal of conducting a rally should be considered and embedded into messages targeting the media as well. It is very beneficial for an advocacy team to successfully persuade the media to promote their campaign at no cost because the reach media advertising has can be considerable.

Promotion is important for an advocacy team because the success of an advocacy effort is largely dependent on the support of many people. When there are many people rooting for the campaign, and when the media broadcast the advocacy campaign, legislators may be more compelled to consider the advocacy message and take action in favor of it. In order to gain the support of people, an advocacy team has to actively promote its campaign, and this can be done through a rally, social media such as Facebook or Twitter, and advertising on radio or television. If the advocacy team wants to have free promotion on radio and television, the team has to use the messaging strategies described in Chapter 6 to persuade the media into providing free news coverage for its campaign.

Pre-Test Draft Advocacy Messages

After developing advocacy messages that incorporate marketing mix concepts and the five key elements described in Chapter 6, the messages need to undergo a pre-test. At this stage, messages are drafts and not yet complete. Pre-testing messages involves an appraisal of which messages and/or message elements work and which do not. Pre-testing messages allows an advocacy team to rectify content and stylistic issues before disseminating the messages to target audiences. Also, it allows an advocacy team to anticipate and prepare for the kind of responses target audiences may have. Pre-testing usually is conducted in a focus group setting, and messages are revised based on feedback from members of the focus groups.

A focus group is a small gathering of homogeneous people assembled by an individual who is seeking more information for a specific inquiry (see

Guest, Namey, & Mitchell, 2013). The people gathered in this setting often are referred to as participants, and their role in the focus group is to provide their opinions to the person inquiring. Although there is no definite number of participants recommended for a focus group, an approximate number of participants ranges from eight to twelve individuals per focus group session (see Guest et al., 2013). As a guide, there should not be too many participants such that some participants contribute very little, and there should not be too few participants because more people will likely share more opinions and a variety of viewpoints. There should be multiple sessions of focus groups with different target audience participants, and like the number of participants, the number of sessions also is not prescribed. When the opinions shared by participants become redundant, the number of focus group sessions is adequate. In other words, conducting additional focus group sessions may end if the responses generated suffice and further inquisition may likely reproduce the same kind of responses. Typically the number of focus group sessions for a topic is approximately three to five per target audience.

The focus group participants assembled by an advocacy team should be representative of the target audiences. As mentioned in Chapter 5, the target audiences of advocacy messages often are legislators, individuals who may be directly or indirectly affected by the advocated health issue, and the media. Therefore, participants of the focus groups should be representative of members of these targeted audiences. For example, if an advocacy team wants to disseminate messages concerning prosthetic parity to people directly or indirectly affected by prosthetic expenses, then participants should involve amputees and their caregivers. If focus group participants in this example are not amputees and do not personally know any amputees, their responses may not be very relevant or beneficial to the advocacy team as they may not be reflective of what the amputee populace experiences. In addition, these participants may become restless and uninvolved in the focus group session. Therefore, an advocacy team should recruit participants for focus group sessions who are representative of the target audiences.

According to Brown, Lindenberger, and Bryant (2008), pre-testing messages should involve formulating communication objectives and asking the participants if the objectives were met. The advocacy team may ask participants if messages are understandable, appealing, relevant, culturally appropriate, credible, and ultimately acceptable and persuasive. After receiving feedback from participants, an advocacy team should revise messages accordingly. If the revisions are substantial, the advocacy team may consider going through another round of pre-testing to assess the revised messages. An advocacy team should continue revisions and pre-testing revised messages until no additional changes are needed or changes are minimal. At that point, the advocacy team should be quite confident that messages are clear and appealing, and the team should be prepared for responses that target audiences may have.

Pre-testing messages is important because it helps avoid costly errors (Brown, Lindenberger, & Bryant, 2008; see also McKenna & Williams, 1993) and also may help anticipate potential confusion. If an advocacy team does not conduct pre-testing and prematurely disseminates messages to target audiences, and the responses do not turn out well or as expected, it may compromise the credibility or future persuasive efforts of the advocacy team. In addition, pre-testing of messages allows the advocacy team to discover aspects of their messages which might not be clear to audiences, thereby preventing potential confusion. Correcting and disseminating messages after bad or unexpected responses from targeted audiences are unnecessarily laborious tasks, which may be avoided with the pre-testing of messages.

Summary

The marketing mix is an important complement to the advocacy messaging process because it helps an advocacy team strategically advocate in a way that is relevant and appealing to audiences. The marketing mix consists of product, price, placement, and promotion. Product refers to the recommended social action (i.e., supporting the advocacy effort) and how it is presented to target audiences. Price refers to the cost incurred by the audience to engage in the social action, and it includes psychological, monetary, energy, or opportunity costs. Place refers to the channel for audiences to support an advocacy effort. Lastly, promotion is the act of bringing the product to the attention of audiences. An advocacy team must incorporate all these components of the marketing mix during the advocacy messaging process in order to advocate strategically and effectively. After developing draft advocacy messages, pre-testing of the messages is necessary for rectifying content and stylistic issues. Pre-testing also helps an advocacy team anticipate and prepare for the kind of responses target audiences may have. After messages are developed and pre-tested, the advocacy team will proceed to Phase 3—Implementation and Evaluation.

References

Albarran, A. B., Anderson, T., Bejar, L. G., Bussart, A. L., Daggett, E., Gibson, S., & … Way, H. (2007). "What happened to our audience?" Radio and new technology uses and gratifications among young adult users. *Journal of Radio Studies, 14*(2), 92–101. doi:10.1080/10955040701583171

Baym, G. (2005). The Daily Show: Discursive integration and the reinvention of political journalism. *Political Communication, 22*(3), 259–276. doi:10.1080/10584600591006492

boyd, d. m., & Ellison, N. B. (2007). Social network sites: Definition, history, and scholarship. *Journal of Computer-Mediated Communication, 13*(1), 210–230. doi: 10.1111/j.1083–6101. 2007.00393.x

Brown, K. M., Lindenberger, J. H., & Bryant, C. A. (2008). Using pretesting to ensure your messages and materials are on strategy. *Health Promotion Practice, 9*(2), 116–122. doi: 10.1177/1524839908315134

Buehner, T. M. (2011). College student preferences for trendy versus classic typefaces. *Operant Subjectivity: The International Journal of Q Methodology, 35*(1), 1–36. Retrieved from http://operantsubjectivity.org/os/about

Burch, E. E., & Henry, W. R. (1974). Opportunity and incremental cost: Attempt to define in systems terms: A comment. *Accounting Review, 49*(1), 118–123. Retrieved from http://aaahq.org/

Caers, R., De Feyter, T., De Couck, M., Stough, T., Vigna, C., & Du Bois, C. (2013). Facebook: A literature review. *New Media & Society, 15*(6), 982–1002. doi: 10.1177/1461444813488061

Caulfield, T., & Bubela, T. (2004). Media representations of genetic discoveries: Hype in the headlines? *Health Law Review, 12*(2), 53–61. Retrieved from http://www.hli.ualberta.ca/

Dibben, N., & Williamson, V. J. (2007). An exploratory survey of in-vehicle music listening. *Psychology of Music, 35*(4), 571–589. doi: 10.1177/0305735607079725

Earl, J. (2006). Pursuing social change online: The use of four protest tactics on the Internet. *Social Science Computer Review, 24*(3), 362–377. doi: 10.1177/0894439305284627

Farrelly, M. C., Hussin, A., & Bauer, U. E. (2007). Effectiveness and cost effectiveness of television, radio and print advertisements in promoting the New York smokers' quitline. *Tobacco Control, 16*(Suppl 1), i21–i23. doi: 10.1136/tc.2007.019984

Gimpel, J. G., & Schuknecht, J. E. (2003). Political participation and the accessibility of the ballot box. *Political Geography, 22*(5), 471–488. doi: 10.1016/S0962–6298(03)00029–5

Grabe, M., Zhou, S., & Barnett, B. (2001). Explicating sensationalism in television news: Content and the bells and whistles of form. *Journal of Broadcasting & Electronic Media, 45*(4), 635–655. doi: 10.1207/s15506878jobem4504_6

Guest, G., Namey, E. E., & Mitchell, M. L. (2013). *Collecting qualitative data: A field manual for applied research.* Thousand Oaks, CA: Sage.

Junco, R., Elavsky, C. M., & Heiberger, G. (2013). Putting Twitter to the test: Assessing outcomes for student collaboration, engagement and success. *British Journal of Educational Technology, 44*(2), 273–287. doi: 10.1111/j.1467–8535.2012.01284.x

Kaplan, A. M., & Haenlein, M. (2010). Users of the world, unite! The challenges and opportunities of social media. *Business horizons*, 53(1), 59–68. doi: 10.1016/j.bushor.2009.09.003

Kotler, P., & Zaltman, G. (1971). Social marketing: An approach to planned social change. *Journal of Marketing*, 35(3), 3–12. Retrieved from http://www.jstor.org/stable/1249783

Kristofferson, K., White, K., & Peloza, J. (2014). The nature of slacktivism: How the social observability of an initial act of token support affects subsequent prosocial action. *Journal of Consumer Research*, 40(6), 1149–1166. doi: 10.1086/674137

Mattson, M. (2010). Health advocacy by accident and discipline. *Health Communication*, 25(6–7), 622–624. doi: 10.1080/10410236.2010.496844

McKenna, J. W., & Williams, K. N. (1993). Crafting effective tobacco counteradvertisements: Lessons from a failed campaign directed at teenagers. *Public Health Reports*, 108, 85. Retrieved from http://www.ncbi.nlm.nih.gov/

Merry, M. K. (2010). Blogging and environmental advocacy: A new way to engage the public?. *Review of Policy Research*, 27(5), 641–656. doi: 10.1111/j.1541–1338.2010.00463.x

Morozov, E. (2012). *The net delusion: The dark side of Internet freedom*. New York: PublicAffairs.

Panagiotopoulos, P., Sams, S., Elliman, T., & Fitzgerald, G. (2011). Do social networking groups support online petitions?. *Transforming Government: People, Process and Policy*, 5(1), 20–31. doi: 10.1108/17506161111114626

Quintelier, E. (2007). Differences in political participation between young and old people. *Contemporary Politics*, 13(2), 165–180. doi:10.1080/13569770701562658

Stephenson, M. T. (2003). Mass media strategies targeting high sensation seekers: What works and why. *American Journal of Health Behavior*, 27(Supplement 3), S233-S238. Retrieved from http://www.ajhb.org/

Xie, B., & Jaeger, P. (2008). Older adults and political participation on the Internet: A cross-cultural comparison of the USA and China. *Journal of Cross-Cultural Gerontology*, 23(1), 1–15. doi: 10.1007/s10823–007–9050–6

· 8 ·

IMPLEMENTATION AND EVALUATION

After an advocacy team has developed advocacy messages and pre-tested those messages, the team proceeds to implement their strategy. Specifically, the team will disseminate the advocacy messages to target audiences. There are several ways to disseminate advocacy messages effectively to target audiences, and some approaches may be more effective for a particular audience than other approaches. The media, relevant populations, and legislators may each respond differently to the advocacy messages. Therefore, the advocacy team will monitor the advocacy process and evaluate any aspect of the strategy that did not work well. As the advocacy campaign nears its end, the advocacy team will evaluate the outcomes and determine the next course of action.

Disseminate Advocacy Messages to Target Audiences

There are several ways to disseminate advocacy messages to target audiences. However, not every approach is suitable for all audiences; depending on who the audience is, various approaches to disseminating messages may be more effective than other approaches. A rally is an effective approach for disseminating advocacy messages to the media; the use of media and promotional talks in communities are effective for communicating advocacy messages to relevant populations; and the use of media and a rally are useful for disseminating advocacy messages to legislators. This is not an exhaustive list of approaches, but these are effective approaches that we recommend.

Disseminating Advocacy Messages to the Media

A rally involves many people convening together to raise awareness about a particular issue. A rally typically involves the use of banners, signboards, and loudspeakers so that the rally may get the attention of onlookers. A rally is effective for disseminating advocacy messages to the media because a rally often catches the attention of the media. Because most media favor sensationalistic approaches to covering news (see e.g., Caulfield & Bubela, 2004; Grabe, Zhou, & Barnett, 2001), a rally is likely to be considered newsworthy by the media. For example, a rally that has many people holding signboards and loudly demanding affordable healthcare outside a state capital may likely be the kind of sensationalistic event the media will report. An advocacy team should use the messaging strategies in Chapter 6 to construct advocacy messages for the rally that will capture the media's attention. These strategies may include the use of bright colors, striking imagery, and slogans, among others.

An advocacy team also should notify the media beforehand that the team will be staging a rally, and brief the media crucial details such as time, location, and the purpose of the rally. It is important not to inundate the media initially with too much health-related information because the media may find the information excessive and uninteresting and consequently find the rally less appealing. An advocacy team should wait for the media to initiate an inquiry for more information before the team gives more information about the health issue. When the media are attracted to an advocacy team's rally and want information about the rally in order to report it, an advocacy team can seize the opportunity to inform the media about the health issue in greater detail. The advocacy team associated with the Indiana Amputee Insurance Protection Coalition is an example of a campaign that received media attention through staging a rally at the statehouse. Through the advocacy team's prompting, several amputees convened and rallied for prosthetic parity on a snowy day in winter. A news reporter who was at the same location to report on another issue saw this interesting arrangement and approached the advocacy team. The news reporter asked the advocacy team for more information regarding their advocacy campaign and proceeded to report on the rally and the issue of prosthetic parity.

There are other ways besides a rally that an advocacy team may use to disseminate advocacy messages to the media, but those approaches may not be as effective. For instance, a press release, phone calls, and emails may be very convenient and efficient approaches and may reach many media outlets in a short span of time, but because the media often have many phone calls and emails to attend to, the media may not invest the time and effort to consider and understand the advocacy team's message. Also, phone calls and emails alone may not be exciting enough to persuade the media to cover the advocacy campaign as news. For these reasons, a rally is recommended for communicating advocacy messages to the media.

Disseminating Advocacy Messages to Relevant Populations

The use of media and promotional talks in communities is effective for disseminating advocacy messages to relevant populations. If an advocacy team manages to get support from the media or pays for advertising to broadcast through the media, the team may spread its advocacy messages to relevant populations through wide-reaching channels such as television news or the radio. Traditional media such as television news and the radio are useful for disseminating advocacy messages because these channels have large viewership/listenership. Despite challenges from newer media (see e.g., Albarran et al., 2007), radio and television news still have a significant number of audiences. For example, many individuals still listen to the radio when they drive a car or truck (Dibben & Williamson, 2007). Television news also has competition from other platforms such as online news and satire news (see e.g., Baym, 2005), but television news still remains the most popular choice for news (Papathanassopoulos et al., 2013). Therefore, traditional media have significant audience numbers and the wide reach enables effective dissemination of advocacy messages. Without the assistance of the media, dissemination of advocacy messages may be difficult. The media may promote advocacy messages to thousands of people with a single advertisement, but without the media an advocacy team may take a much longer time and need greater effort to attain the same dissemination results. Using the media to communicate to audiences also is beneficial because an advocacy campaign that is reported on media outlets such as television news may seem more legitimate, serious, and urgent (Wallack & Dorfman, 1996).

However, there may be a downside in using the media to disseminate advocacy messages; because the media broadcasts information to a mass audience, the advocacy messages also may be communicated to people outside of relevant populations. For example, if an advocacy message regarding prosthetic parity is broadcast on television, the message may be received by people who are not directly or indirectly affected by prosthetic issues. This inclusion of people outside of relevant populations should not pose a problem though; the people outside of relevant populations likely will disregard the message while relevant populations may attend to the message. However, it is unknown whether the proportion of relevant populations in relation to the mass audience is large, moderate, or small. For example, a television news report about prosthetic parity may have 100,000 viewers but only 30 of those viewers may be amputees or caregivers of amputees. In such a situation, the media may not be effective in disseminating advocacy messages to relevant populations. Although there are these possible concerns in using the media to disseminate advocacy messages, it should be emphasized that such concerns are only a possibility; in other words, overall, it is unlikely that the media will be ineffective in communicating to relevant populations. Therefore, an advocacy team should use the media to disseminate advocacy messages whenever possible. An advocacy team can also use other approaches in order to be more certain that advocacy messages are disseminated to relevant populations. Conducting promotional talks in communities is one such approach.

Promotional talks in communities involve an advocacy team speaking about the advocacy campaign or health issue in communities that are likely to have relevant audiences. For example, if the advocated health issue is related to cancer, an advocacy team may conduct the promotional talks in a region where there is a greater distribution of cancer patients. In order to find out which location has a greater distribution of cancer patients, an advocacy team may use the research strategies described in Chapter 5. For example, an advocacy team advocating for cancer-related issues may use scholarly articles that inform readers about the distribution of cancer and conduct promotional talks in the region with the highest distribution. Communities may not only refer to regions (e.g., county, towns, etc.) but also to specific gathering places such as cancer support communities, facilities for cancer support groups, and so on. These gathering places often have the most relevant audiences because people directly and indirectly affected by a particular health issue convene in those places. A good method that an advocacy team may use to find these gathering places is the community asset mapping technique discussed in Chapter 4. An advocacy team may interview residents of a community or scout around the community in order to locate those gathering places. When the community or gathering place is found, an advocacy team may request to conduct its promotional presentations.

Promotional talks are meant to be more personalized than media messages in bringing about awareness of the advocacy campaign and advocated health issue. These talks should include an explanation of what the advocacy campaign is about, what the advocated health issue is, how the health issue affects the audience, and how the audience may support the advocacy campaign. It is important for an advocacy team to use the messaging strategies described in Chapter 6 to design effective and attractive promotional talks. By not using these strategies, audiences in those communities may not be interested in hearing the promotional talks. As an example of messaging strategies for promotional talks, an advocacy team may use banners with bright colors to attract audience's attention and use emotional appeals to compel the audience to support the advocacy campaign. As with all persuasive messages, the promotional talks should inform the audience about the advocacy campaign and health issue, but should not inundate the audience with excessive information. It also is important for the advocacy team to provide its contact information to the audience and to get contact information from the audience members. Sometimes, the latter may not be possible because the audience may not be willing to share their contact details. Therefore, a promotional talk should be persuasive and the team must appear trustworthy so that the audience may feel comfortable sharing contact information. Contact information usually includes emails or phone numbers, and such information is important because it allows for direct communication with relevant populations. An advocacy team should not ask for contact information such as home addresses because the audience may perceive such a request as being too invasive or inappropriate. Promotional talks are useful for communicating to a specific audience such as relevant populations and should be adopted in conjunction with the use of media.

Other approaches for disseminating advocacy messages to relevant audiences may not work as well as the approaches just described. For instance, an advocacy team may rely solely on sending out pamphlets to disseminate advocacy messages to relevant audiences, but such an approach may not be most effective. It should be stressed that this does not mean that sending out pamphlets should not be considered for reaching out to relevant populations; it simply means that such approaches may not be as effective. For example, advocacy pamphlets have to compete with many other pamphlets and mailings and therefore are unlikely to be attended to by relevant audience members. Another approach that may not be as effective in disseminating advocacy messages to relevant populations is cold calling, which refers to the process of randomly calling people. Cold calls are not as effective because people may be skeptical and therefore become unresponsive to messages. In summary, an advocacy team may use a variety of approaches including cold calls and sending pamphlets, but these approaches may be less effective than the other recommended approaches including the media and promotional talks.

Disseminating Advocacy Messages to Legislators

The use of media and rallies is effective for communicating advocacy messages to legislators. Because legislators are responsible for the welfare of their constituents, media reports about an alarming health issue and a health advocacy campaign associated with that issue may capture the attention of legislators. Alarming health issues imply that the welfare of a community is wanting, and therefore it behooves legislators to respond to those health issues and the associated advocacy campaigns. Furthermore, media reports on alarming health issues and associated advocacy campaigns may effectively capture the attention of legislators because they realize that many of their constituents will have seen those reports. For example, if the news reports that health advocates are demanding policy changes because cancer treatment is unaffordable, constituents who receive such news may feel that their legislators should implement policy changes, and consequently legislators may be compelled to address those potential policy changes.

In addition to traditional media such as television news and newspapers, social media can complement effective communication of advocacy messages to legislators. Social networking websites and social media applications can be useful for promoting awareness of an advocated health issue to many people (see Chapter 7). For example, an advocacy team may use web logs (i.e., blogs) to inform audiences about the health issue and associated advocacy campaign or direct audiences to links to online news reporting about the health issue and the campaign. These blogs may increase awareness among constituents and further compel legislators to take notice of the advocacy campaign. Furthermore, legislators may view those blogs if they want to obtain more information about the health issue and associated advocacy campaign.

A rally also is an effective approach to communicate advocacy messages to legislators. In particular, a rally conducted outside a state capitol may be very effective. It is difficult for legislators to miss advocacy messages if those messages are presented in front of the building where they work. The pressure on legislators to heed advocacy messages may be increased if the media reports on a rally conducted outside the state capitol building. A rally should be as attention-grabbing as possible to attract the attention of legislators. For example, a rally could have banners, signboards, and loudspeakers so that advocacy messages may be brought across both visually and audibly. Rally participants also may be particularly vocal when legislators walk into or out of the building, as that usually catches their attention.

It should be noted that our recommendation of such approaches does not mean that the support of relevant populations is not important in communicating with legislators; these recommended approaches are founded upon the support of relevant populations. For example, a media report on a rally is not as effective as a media report on a rally that has strong support from the local community. Also, a rally is more effective if local constituents are participating in the rally. Therefore, support from relevant populations should be the driving force behind the successful use of the media and a rally for disseminating health advocacy messages to legislators.

In sum, certain approaches are more effective than others in disseminating advocacy messages to target audiences. A rally typically works well for disseminating health advocacy messages to the media; the use of media and promotional talks in communities also is effective for disseminating advocacy messages to relevant populations; and media use and a rally are important for communicating advocacy messages to legislators. The media, relevant populations, and legislators may each respond differently to the advocacy messages. Therefore, an advocacy team needs to monitor and evaluate the performance of the team's strategy and advocacy process.

Process Evaluation

The media, relevant populations, and legislators may react favorably or unfavorably to an advocacy team's strategy and advocacy messages. An advocacy team should monitor and evaluate the performance of the team's strategy and advocacy process so that the team may rectify aspects of its campaign that did not work well. Because the media, relevant populations, and legislators may react favorably or unfavorably to the advocacy strategy and messages, the advocacy team should be sure to respond accordingly.

Evaluating Process with the Media

The media may react favorably to the advocacy strategy and messages by supporting an advocacy campaign. A news media may offer to provide news coverage for an advocacy campaign, while other forms of media may offer to provide free advertising between programs. When such favorable opportunities arise, an advocacy team should provide the media with more details about the health issue and associated advocacy campaign. It is unlikely that the media will know about the health issue thoroughly before the advocacy team provides an explication of the issue; therefore an advocacy team should provide more information. Giving more details about the advocated health issue to the media is necessary because an advocacy team would not want the media to provide inaccurate information or incorrectly portray the campaign.

On the other hand, the media may react unfavorably to the advocacy strategy and messages. The media may react unfavorably by declining to promote the advocacy campaign. In such a situation, an advocacy team may want to look at other media outlets that may be more supportive. For example, if the media outlet is a large national news organization and declines to promote the advocacy campaign because the campaign is deemed less important to a national audience than other news, an advocacy team may consider approaching a smaller news organization such as a state news company. Sometimes, media companies decline covering an advocacy campaign because the campaign may not be relevant to the focus of the media company or its target audiences. For example, some magazines that focus on mitigating cancer issues may not want to feature an article on prosthetic parity. Again, in such a situation an advocacy team may consider approaching more relevant media companies.

There may be a rare possibility that the media misrepresent an advocacy campaign. Because many media outlets adopt sensationalistic approaches (see e.g., Caulfield & Bubela, 2004; Grabe et al., 2001), there may be a possibility that some media may intentionally exaggerate or misrepresent an advocacy campaign. For example, instead of a depicting an advocacy rally as a well-organized activity for social justice, some media may portray the rally as a group of rancorous and rebellious people. Intentional misrepresentation may occur in media's emphasis on sensationalistic aspects of advocacy. Some media may deliberately focus more on sensationalistic aspects such as the experiences of people with a health issue instead of informing audiences about how they may support an advocacy campaign. In such a situation an advocacy team may want to approach other media companies that would promote the health advocacy campaign more comprehensively. Usually, media that are more academic, such as healthcare magazines or documentary channels, are more accurate with reporting and less sensationalistic. However, the drawback is that these more academic media outlets often have smaller audiences and, as a result, fewer people may be informed about the health issue and the advocacy campaign. An advocacy team may still consider media outlets such as television news companies, but the advocacy team should be extra deliberate about having accurate information presented. All in all, an advocacy team should be careful with the media organizations they interact with. Also, the team should consistently uphold strong standards so that misrepresentation would be difficult to achieve.

Evaluating Process with Relevant Populations

An advocacy team may interact with some members of relevant populations through emails, phone calls, or community talks to gauge how relevant populations are responding to the advocacy process. The interactions should be brief and casual, and a few of such interactions should provide a sense of how relevant populations are responding to the advocacy process. The number of interactions depends on saturation (see Chapter 4), during which responses from additional interactions repeat previous responses, are predictable, and do not provide new information. These interactions not only should be with people in a particular area, but with individuals across different areas or demographics. For example, if advocacy messages are disseminated throughout the state of Indiana, an advocacy team should not merely interact with members of relevant populations in the city of Fort Wayne to get a sense of how relevant populations are reacting to the advocacy process. Instead, the advocacy team also should make inquiries with people from other areas within Indiana, such as the cities of Lafayette, West Lafayette, Indianapolis, and so on. Limiting inquiry to just one area of the state, such as Fort Wayne, would provide a gauge of how relevant populations in Fort Wayne are responding; it may not accurately reflect how people in other parts of the state are responding. By inquiring from members of relevant populations across different areas, the advocacy team may get a more accurate sense of how relevant populations are reacting to the advocacy process.

Besides geographical considerations, an advocacy team also should interact with members of relevant populations from different demographics. For example, if an advocacy team is campaigning for cancer-related issues, the advocacy team should interact not only with adults, but with the elderly and youth as well. If an advocacy team does not inquire with people of other demographics, an advocacy team will be remiss in gathering both the positive and negative reactions of others toward the advocacy process. For instance, the elderly may dislike the notion of online petitions in advocacy messages because the elderly may not like to use online channels for political activity (see e.g., Xie & Jaeger, 2008). Other demographics that an advocacy team should consider are sex, race, and socioeconomic status, among others. An advocacy team should contact some members of relevant populations across areas and demographics in order to get a sense of whether relevant populations are responding favorably or unfavorably to the advocacy process.

Relevant populations may react favorably to an advocacy process by wanting to show their support for an advocacy campaign. In such a situation an advocacy team must make sure that there are ample details regarding how relevant populations may support a campaign. For example, if a team uses online petitions, there should be adequate directions for relevant populations to know where and how to sign the petitions online. An advocacy team also should assess the level of support across different geographical areas or demographics. For example, if advocacy messages are disseminated throughout the state of Indiana, certain locations, such as the state's largest city, Indianapolis, may have a greater number of supporters from relevant populations in comparison to smaller locations such as Lafayette and Fort Wayne. An advocacy team should collect this information so that the team can, as accurately as possible, evaluate the outcome of the campaign.

Relevant populations may react unfavorably to an advocacy process by declining to support an advocacy campaign. Because health advocacy campaigns often involve health concerns and rarely stir controversy, it is unlikely for relevant populations to react hostilely to advocacy messages. However, relevant populations may disregard or reject advocacy messages if they respond unfavorably to the messages. Relevant populations may disregard or reject advocacy messages if they feel that the messages do not address the health concern adequately or are asking for too much commitment on their part. For example, relevant populations may reject an advocacy message that asks them to participate in five consecutive days of rallying outside a state capitol. Although five consecutive days of rallying may be effective, such a request may be considered too demanding for relevant populations. Relevant populations also may disregard advocacy messages that fail to be impactful. For example, advocacy messages that do not address the susceptibility of relevant populations to a health issue and do not motivate audiences to take action are unlikely to have impact and are likely to be disregarded by relevant populations. An advocacy team should monitor for such reactions and record them so that the team may rectify aspects of advocacy messages that did not work well later.

Evaluating Process with Legislators

Legislators may respond favorably to an advocacy process by voting for the advocated bill to pass. To check progress with legislators, an advocacy team's lobbyist or team members may contact legislators or other politicians to get a sense of how legislators are responding to the messages. Of all the target audiences, the reactions of legislators are most vital because favorable responses likely may lead to policy change in favor of the health advocacy campaign's efforts. However, it should be emphasized that favorable responses from the media and relevant populations should not be overlooked because their responses contribute greatly to how legislators react.

Legislators may respond unfavorably to an advocacy process by voting against the advocated bill. The advocacy team's lobbyist should find out why legislators were not in favor of the bill so that the team may correct their strategy in future advocacy efforts. Legislators also may respond unfavorably by deeming that voting action is not required for the advocated issue. Such circumstances may occur if the advocacy messages for legislators did not have enough impact. For instance, advocacy messages may have failed to mention that the campaign has garnered a lot of support from constituents within the state. Or, the advocacy messages may not have been communicated through effective channels, such as the media or a rally. Ineffective channels may cause legislators to perceive the advocated issue as being less serious, urgent, or supported than it actually may be. For example, in contrast to the use of television news, communicating an advocated health issue through a lobbyist alone may not give the perception that a community is aware of the health issue and that many people are supporting policy change. The advocacy team needs to keep a record of why legislators responded unfavorably so that the team may correct their strategy and advocacy messages for future advocacy efforts.

Outcome Evaluation

An advocacy process is completed when all target audiences have responded to an advocacy team's strategy and advocacy messages. During this stage, an advocacy team should evaluate the outcome of the campaign and determine the next action to take. There are two possible outcomes: the advocacy campaign was successful or the campaign was unsuccessful.

Whether an advocacy campaign was successful or not depends largely on the interpretation of the advocacy team. For example, advocacy groups that campaigned against smoking in airplanes in 1972 could have interpreted the implementation of separate sections for smokers and non-smokers as a success. Alternatively, those advocacy groups could have interpreted it as not yet successful and resumed advocacy, which they did (Holm & Davis, 2004). A more precise way to determine whether a campaign was successful is to compare the advocacy result with the position statement described in Chapter 3. To recap, the position statement contains both the stance of the advocacy team regarding the health concern and the goal of the team. If the advocacy result is similar to the position statement, the advocacy campaign is successful, and vice versa. To illustrate, in 2004, the National African American Tobacco Prevention Network launched an effort to abolish Kool (i.e., their position statement), a flavored cigarette that targeted African American youth. The network was able to abolish Kool and was awarded $1.4 million in a legal settlement (i.e., results) (Freudenberg, Bradley, & Serrano, 2009). In this illustration, the result was consistent with the network's position statement (i.e., abolishing Kool). Therefore, the network likely would determine that their campaign was successful. If Kool continued to be available for purchase, the result would have been dissimilar from the network's position statement and the network likely would have determined their campaign was unsuccessful. Depending on the campaign outcome (i.e., successful or unsuccessful), an advocacy team needs to take appropriate future actions.

If an advocacy campaign is determined to be successful, the advocacy team may conclude the campaign by informing relevant populations regarding the policy changes implemented or the progress that was achieved. It is vital to inform as many relevant populations as possible because they are the ones who are most positively affected by the policy changes. An advocacy team may inform relevant populations through several ways, including social media, which is useful for such a task because it can disseminate and exchange large amounts of information rapidly (Lovejoy, Waters, & Saxton, 2012). However, an advocacy team should be mindful of factors that may prevent such information from reaching relevant populations, such as lack of Internet access. To circumvent such a problem, an advocacy team may communicate information through alternative channels such as magazines or phone calls (Kratzke, Wilson, & Vilchis, 2013). However, such outlets often are more costly to use than new media (Pickerill, 2001). Kratzke and colleagues (2013) posited that technological disparity is decreasing for mobile phones and that the prevalence of mobile phone usage and text messaging among rural women was similar to the national average in the United States. Calling relevant populations may be an option, but such an approach is costly (Link, Battaglia, Frankel, Osborn, & Mokdad, 2007) and rather impractical because there may be too many people to call. Therefore, after reviewing literature on information dissemination, the use of social media seems to be the optimal approach for informing relevant populations because it is the most cost-effective and wide-reaching approach (see Lovejoy et al., 2012; Pickerill, 2001). An advocacy team generally should inform relevant populations through social media and accommodate accordingly for those who lack access.

If an advocacy campaign is determined to be unsuccessful, the advocacy team can either continue with its advocacy effort or withdraw from advocacy. If the former decision is made, an advocacy team should identify the strengths and weaknesses of their campaign so that the team may correct aspects of the campaign that did not work well and improve the team's strategy for continuing its advocacy effort. The next chapter (Chapter 9) will elaborate on this scenario. If the latter decision is made, the advocacy team should conclude the campaign by informing relevant populations about any progress the campaign made. An advocacy team may decide to withdraw the campaign because there were insufficient resources to continue, a stalemate was reached and further action is not possible or needed, policy change is not possible, or because the team prefers to withdraw. It should be stressed that there always is progress to inform relevant populations about, even in the face of ostensible loss. For example, an advocacy campaign likely will have promoted awareness concerning the advocated health issue (e.g., Freudenberg et al., 2009) and that is progress. Also, advocacy campaigns that were unsuccessful also should be documented so that other advocates and campaign scholars may learn from those campaigns (e.g., Pless, 2007).

Summary

An advocacy team that has developed and pre-tested its advocacy messages will proceed to implement its strategy and disseminate its messages. There are various approaches to disseminating advocacy messages, and certain approaches are more effective for particular target audiences than other approaches. A rally is an effective approach for disseminating advocacy messages to the media; media use and promotional talks in communities are effective for disseminating advocacy messages to relevant populations; and media use and a rally are useful for communicating advocacy messages to legislators. The media, relevant populations, and legislators may each respond differently to the advocacy process, and therefore an advocacy team needs to evaluate the responses of target audiences and react accordingly. An advocacy process is completed when target audiences have responded to an advocacy team's strategy and advocacy messages. An advocacy team will need to assess the outcome and determine if the team's campaign was successful or unsuccessful. If the campaign was successful or if the advocacy team decides to withdraw from further advocacy efforts, the advocacy team should inform relevant populations about the policy changes or other progress made. If the advocacy team determines that the campaign was unsuccessful, but wants to continue their efforts, the team will proceed to the Correction Loop. The Correction Loop is discussed in the next chapter.

References

Albarran, A. B., Anderson, T., Bejar, L. G., Bussart, A. L., Daggett, E., Gibson, S., & ... Way, H. (2007). "What happened to our audience?" Radio and new technology uses and gratifications among young adult users. *Journal of Radio Studies, 14*(2), 92–101. doi:10.1080/10955040701583171

Baym, G. (2005). The Daily Show: Discursive integration and the reinvention of political journalism. *Political Communication, 22*(3), 259–276. doi:10.1080/10584600591006492

Caulfield, T., & Bubela, T. (2004). Media representations of genetic discoveries: Hype in the headlines?. *Health Law Review, 12*(2), 53–61. Retrieved from http://www.hli.ualberta.ca/

Dibben, N., & Williamson, V. J. (2007). An exploratory survey of in-vehicle music listening. *Psychology of Music, 35*(4), 571–589. doi: 10.1177/0305735607079725

Freudenberg, N., Bradley, S. P., & Serrano, M. (2009). Public health campaigns to change industry practices that damage health: An analysis of 12 case studies. *Health Education & Behavior, 36*(2), 230–249. doi: 10.1177/1090198107301330

Grabe, M., Zhou, S., & Barnett, B. (2001). Explicating sensationalism in television news: Content and the bells and whistles of form. *Journal of Broadcasting & Electronic Media*, 45(4), 635–655. doi: 10.1207/s15506878jobem4504_6

Holm, A. L., & Davis, R. M. (2004). Clearing the airways: Advocacy and regulation for smoke-free airlines. *Tobacco Control*, 13(suppl 1), i30–i36. doi: 10.1136/tc.2003.005686

Kratzke, C., Wilson, S., & Vilchis, H. (2013). Reaching rural women: Breast cancer prevention information seeking behaviors and interest in internet, cell phone, and text use. *Journal of Community Health*, 38(1), 54–61. doi: 10.1007/s10900–012–9579–3

Link, M. W., Battaglia, M. P., Frankel, M. R., Osborn, L., & Mokdad, A. H. (2007). Reaching the U.S. cell phone generation. *Public Opinion Quarterly*, 71(5), 814–839. doi: 10.1093/poq/nfm051

Lovejoy, K., Waters, R. D., & Saxton, G. D. (2012). Engaging stakeholders through Twitter: How nonprofit organizations are getting more out of 140 characters or less. *Public Relations Review*, 38(2), 313–318. doi: 10.1016/j.pubrev.2012.01.005

Papathanassopoulos, S., Coen, S., Curran, J., Aalberg, T., Rowe, D., Jones, P., ... & Tiffen, R. (2013). Online threat, but television is still dominant: A comparative study of 11 nations' news consumption. *Journalism Practice*, 7(6), 690–704. doi: 10.1080/17512786.2012.761324

Pickerill, J. (2001). Environmental internet activism in Britain. *Peace Review*, 13(3), 365–370. doi:10.1080/13668800120079063

Pless, I. B. (2007). A chronology of failed advocacy and frustration. *Injury Prevention*, 13(2), 73–74. doi: 10.1136/ip. 2007.015776

Wallack, L., & Dorfman, L. (1996). Media advocacy: A strategy for advancing policy and promoting health. *Health Education & Behavior*, 23(3), 293–317. doi: 10.1177/109019819602300303

Xie, B., & Jaeger, P. (2008). Older adults and political participation on the internet: A cross-cultural comparison of the USA and China. *Journal of Cross-Cultural Gerontology*, 23(1), 1–15. doi: 10.1007/s10823–007–9050–6

· 9 ·

CORRECTION LOOP

After an advocacy team implements its strategy, disseminates advocacy messages, and evaluates the advocacy process and outcome, the team will determine whether the advocacy campaign was successful or not. If the campaign was unsuccessful and the advocacy team decides to resume the advocacy effort, the advocacy team will need to go through the Correction Loop. The Correction Loop is a phase during which an advocacy team cycles back to Phase 2 (i.e., formative research and message development) and Phase 3 (i.e., implementation and evaluation). In short, an advocacy team will have to correct its strategy and advocacy messages based on the process and outcome evaluations. There are two factors to consider in correcting strategy: reasons for negative responses and geographical or demographical differences.

Reasons for Negative Responses

In order to identify reasons for negative responses toward advocacy messages, an advocacy team may conduct surveys, interviews, or focus group sessions (refer to Chapter 4 for how to conduct methods). There are several possible reasons for negative responses toward advocacy messages. An advocacy team should identify the reasons for negative responses and correct the team's strategy and revise advocacy messages accordingly. Although not exhaustive, these are possible reasons: lack of information, participation apprehension, and/or advocacy messages were not convincing enough.

Lack of Information

Negative responses toward advocacy messages may have been due to a lack of information in advocacy messages. For example, advocacy messages may not have had adequate information regarding the advocated health issue. Consequently, audiences may not have comprehended the significance of the health issue and were likely unmotivated to support the advocacy effort. There are various types of information that are necessary in advocacy messages and the exclusion of or an inadequate amount of such information may have resulted in the negative responses from audiences. This information may include: steps/procedures involved in supporting advocacy, advocacy team's contact information, the advocated health issue, and the consequence of a successful or unsuccessful advocacy campaign.

Steps involved in supporting advocacy were missing or inadequate. Steps/procedures involved in supporting advocacy are important because without such information audiences may not feel equipped for supporting an advocacy effort. This is akin to perceived self-efficacy, which refers to one's belief that he or she knows what to do and has the ability to take action (see Bandura, 1990; Moriarty & Stryker, 2008). For example, if an advocacy campaign used an online petition and provided instructions on accessing and signing the online petition, the audiences likely would have felt equipped to support the advocacy campaign. In contrast, audiences who were not provided the website address to the online petition or not given instructions on how to sign the petition likely would have felt unequipped to support the advocacy campaign. Consequently, audiences who felt unequipped likely may have responded negatively to advocacy messages by not supporting the advocacy campaign. If an advocacy team discovers that instructions for supporting the advocacy campaign were missing or inadequate, the team should add clear and concise instructions in the revised advocacy messages. It is stressed that instructions should be concise because excessive instructional information may distract audiences from the main message (e.g., the advocated health issue). Also, excessive instructional information may overwhelm audiences and may give audiences the impression that supporting an advocacy campaign involves tedious or complicated steps. If supporting an advocacy campaign truly involved many steps/procedures, an advocacy team may consider implementing a different approach for audiences to support the advocacy campaign. For instance, instead of asking audiences to write and send a personal email to the legislation office, an advocacy team could simply ask audiences to sign an online petition.

Advocacy team's contact information was missing. An advocacy team's contact information is necessary because without it audiences may be skeptical or may not know who to contact for advocacy-related concerns. Audiences may be skeptical when there is no contact information available because the lack of identification may seem unprofessional or suspicious. Most professional organizations have contact information available in promotional messages or on the organization's website. Therefore, advocacy messages that omit contact information likely would seem unprofessional. Also, audiences may have been suspicious of an advocacy campaign that does not have contact information because the campaign may have seemed less legitimate. Skepticism in audiences may have resulted in the negative responses toward advocacy messages (i.e., not supporting the advocacy campaign). If contact information was unavailable, audiences may not have known who to contact for advocacy-related questions and concerns. For example, if contact information was unavailable and audiences wanted to support an advocacy campaign in ways other than signing an online petition, these audiences likely will not have known what alternatives were available. Consequently, the potential support of these audiences likely was lost. An advocacy team that realizes that the team's contact information was missing in advocacy messages should include contact details in the revised messages.

Information regarding advocated health issue was missing or inadequate. Audiences without adequate knowledge about an advocated health issue likely would not have supported an advocacy campaign. Information regarding an advocated health issue may have been missing or inadequate if advocacy messages focused too much on aesthetics or delivery. For example, a video message may have focused too much on depicting accidents, dramatic hospital scenes, emergency room operations, and failed to mention the health issue adequately (e.g., affordable healthcare). An advocacy team that realizes information regarding the advocated health issue was missing or inadequate should incorporate such information in the revised advocacy messages. The advocacy team also should be careful not to provide too much information on the health issue in the revised advocacy messages as that may be considered boring for audiences. As mentioned in Chapter 6, pre-testing is a good technique for gauging audiences' receptivity to advocacy messages. An advocacy team may pre-test the revised advocacy messages to determine if additional information regarding the advocated health issue is insufficient, adequate, or excessive.

Consequences of successful/unsuccessful advocacy campaign were not mentioned. The consequences of a successful or unsuccessful advocacy campaign should have been mentioned in advocacy messages. Such information may motivate audiences to support an advocacy campaign. For example, if audiences knew that the success or failure of an advocacy campaign against targeted food marketing will largely determine if such marketing will continue or cease targeting their children (see Ebbeling, Pawlak, & Ludwig, 2002; Swinburn et al., 2011), the audiences likely would have supported the advocacy campaign. In contrast, if audiences were unaware of the consequences of an advocacy campaign, the audiences likely would have been unconcerned about the campaign and therefore would not support the campaign. Audiences are unlikely to be motivated to process an advocacy message if the perceived threat (e.g., targeted food marketing to children) is low (Witte, 1994). Consequently, audiences may not have been motivated to support an advocacy campaign if information regarding the consequences of an advocacy campaign were not mentioned in advocacy messages. Therefore, if such information was not mentioned or inadequately mentioned in advocacy messages, such information should be elucidated in revised advocacy messages.

Adequate information is necessary for audiences to be certain and confident in supporting an advocacy campaign. A lack of information therefore may have compromised the certainty and confidence of audiences in supporting an advocacy campaign. Although not exhaustive, key information that should be included and adequately addressed is: steps/procedures involved in supporting advocacy, advocacy team's contact information, the advocated health issue, and the consequences of a successful or unsuccessful advocacy campaign. Failure to adequately include this information may have resulted in negative responses toward advocacy messages. Therefore, an advocacy team should include information that was previously lacking in the revised advocacy messages.

Participation Apprehension

Participation apprehension may have been a reason for negative responses toward advocacy messages. As described previously, audiences may have had apprehension about participating in the advocacy campaign because of a lack of information. For instance, if there were inadequate details regarding the advocated health issue, audiences could have been uncertain about what the advocacy cause was and therefore became apprehensive in supporting the advocacy campaign. Besides a lack of information, audiences may have been apprehensive about participating in the advocacy campaign because of concerns about costs involved. These costs may be physical, emotional, financial, responsibilities, and backlashes.

Physical costs. Audiences may have had concerns about the physical efforts required in supporting an advocacy effort. For example, if the suggested approach for supporting an advocacy effort was rallying, audience members may have been concerned about the duration in which they have to stand or walk and hold a signboard. For example, audiences may have imagined that rallying would take about two hours of walking and holding a signboard on a hot day. Such a notion may have been daunting for audiences and, as a result, some audience members may have been apprehensive about supporting an advocacy campaign. If an advocacy team discovers, through surveys or interview, that some audiences had such concerns, an advocacy team may want to change the approach for supporting an advocacy effort to a less physically demanding one. Alternatively, the advocacy team may attempt to convince audiences in revised advocacy messages that the approach for supporting the advocacy effort is not laborious. If the approach for supporting an advocacy campaign did not require much physical effort, but some audiences had a perception otherwise, the revised advocacy messages should clarify to audiences that supporting the advocacy effort would not require much physical effort.

Emotional costs. Audiences may have had concerns about the emotional involvement in supporting an advocacy campaign and were thus apprehensive about supporting the campaign. For example, audiences may not have wanted to experience the disappointment of an unsuccessful advocacy campaign. Such a concern may have arisen if advocacy messages used emotional appeals excessively (see Guttman & Salmon, 2004). To address this concern, an advocacy team will have to revise advocacy messages so that the messages will not be emotionally draining and burdensome for audiences. For example, if a prosthetic parity message excessively depicted the struggles of amputees without prosthetic limbs, audiences may have had misperceived advocacy participation as emotionally burdensome and taxing. Thus, the message would have to be revised to appropriately depict the struggles of amputees.

Financial costs. Audiences may have been concerned about the monetary costs that may be involved in supporting an advocacy campaign. For instance, audiences may have felt that the fuel needed for traveling to a rally would be costly, and thus decided against supporting an advocacy campaign. Audiences also may have considered financial costs in terms of opportunity costs, which is the sacrifice of alternatives due to a decision made (Burch & Henry, 1974). For example, audiences may have thought that the time needed for supporting an advocacy campaign could be used for earning more income instead. If audiences had such concerns about financial costs, an advocacy team will need to emphasize in the revised advocacy messages that the advocacy cause is worth the sacrifices or costs.

Responsibilities involved. Certain audiences may have had concerns about having too many responsibilities in supporting an advocacy campaign and therefore became apprehensive about supporting the campaign. For instance, audiences may have had concerns that once they agree to sign an online petition, they would have to commit to other future requests such as donating to a fundraising event for the advocacy effort. If audiences had such a concern, an advocacy team will need to be clear about the expected responsibilities of supporters in the revised advocacy messages. The expected responsibilities also should not be burdensome for supporters to undertake. Audiences likely may take up greater responsibilities if advocacy messages are persuasive. In other words, if advocacy messages communicate the health issue threat (Witte, 1994), the recommended action, and how audiences can confidently undertake the recommended action (see Witte, 1992) effectively, audiences may be more motivated to take action and therefore may be more willing to take greater responsibilities. For instance, less motivated audiences may only engage in signing an online petition, whereas audiences who perceive the health issue as threatening may want to do more than just sign an online petition, such as rallying. Therefore, an advocacy team may consider focusing on persuasion in revising advocacy messages so that the issue of responsibilities may be a lesser concern.

Backlashes. Although getting into trouble with political authorities may be less common for the public in the United States than other countries (Sedler, 2006), there may be individuals in the United States who have such a concern. Individuals may have a fear that the authorities would track down supporters of an advocacy effort and cause supporters problems in their lives (e.g., career). Typically, American-born audiences may not have this concern, but audiences who are immigrants may have concerns about political involvement, particularly immigrants who had negative experiences with political systems or had limited freedom of speech in other countries. If certain audiences had such a concern, the revised advocacy messages should give audiences the impression or assurance that supporters of the advocacy campaign will not get into trouble with the authorities. For example, the revised messages may emphasize that the advocacy team will protect the identities of supporters as much as possible.

Participation apprehension may have been a reason for negative responses toward advocacy messages. A lack of information regarding the advocacy campaign and concerns about costs involved in supporting the campaign may have resulted in participation apprehension. Specifically, the concerns about costs may have been physical, emotional, financial, responsibilities, and backlashes. An advocacy team needs to ascertain if audiences had such concerns and address those concerns accordingly in the revised advocacy messages.

Advocacy Messages Were Not Convincing Enough

Audiences may have had negative responses toward advocacy messages because these messages were not convincing enough. Advocacy messages may have been unconvincing if there was inadequate information regarding the advocacy campaign. As previously mentioned, inadequate information in advocacy messages may have caused an advocacy campaign to appear unprofessional or suspicious, and therefore the messages likely would not have been convincing. Besides inadequate information, advocacy messages likely were unconvincing if the messages did not seem urgent, had little relevance, or did not employ appeal strategies.

If advocacy messages did not give audiences a sense of urgency, the messages may not have been convincing enough. For example, if advocacy messages did not stress the challenges that many amputees may experience if parity across insurance plans for the coverage of prosthetics is not enforced, audiences may have thought that prosthetic parity was not urgently required and therefore not prioritized supporting the advocacy campaign. As mentioned in Chapter 5, an advocacy team may use news media to enhance audiences' sense of urgency for the advocacy campaign (Wallack & Dorfman, 1996). Besides news media, an advocacy team may emphasize in the revised advocacy messages the need for the advocacy campaign to be successful. The revised advocacy messages also may present alarming statistics concerning the advocated health issue so that the health issue seems pressing. Advocacy messages also may seem urgent if the health issue appears threatening to audiences. Audiences may be more motivated to process messages if the perceived threat is high (Witte, 1994). However, emphasis on threat of the health issue should be accompanied by self-efficacious directions for audiences to support the advocacy campaign (Witte, 1992).

Advocacy messages may not have been convincing if the messages appeared to have little relevance to audiences. For example, advocacy messages may not have seemed relevant if the messages were not culturally relatable. Advocacy messages should be revised to be culturally relatable for audiences so that audience members may pay more attention to the messages and better process the information (see Kreuter & Haughton, 2006; see also Kreuter, Lukwago, Bucholtz, Clark, & Sanders-Thompson, 2003). Some audiences may have felt that advocacy messages were irrelevant because they were unaware about their risk of or susceptibility to the health issue. For example, audiences in a particular region may not have been aware that they had a high risk of cancer and therefore were remiss about advocacy messages related to cancer. There also may have been audiences who knew of the risks of a health issue, but did not believe the health issue would affect them. For example, there may have been individuals who smoked cigarettes, but did not believe that they will ever get lung cancer. In such situations, an advocacy team should include more relevant statistical evidence in the revised advocacy messages. In that way, audiences may become aware of their risk or susceptibility to the health issue and may be more compelled to consider the health issue more seriously. Chapter 5 includes a lengthier discussion of the use of statistical evidence.

Advocacy messages also may not have been convincing because appeal strategies were not used or were used ineffectively. For example, if messages lacked guilt appeals (Coulter, Cotte, & Moore, 1999), audiences may not have been compelled to support an advocacy campaign. For instance, if audiences were not informed that their inaction would cause, say, prosthetic limbs to remain unaffordable for amputees, those audiences may not see the urgency of prosthetic parity and thus not support the campaign. If appeal strategies were not used or were used ineffectively, the revised advocacy messages should use the appeal strategies described in Chapter 6.

Audiences may have reacted negatively to advocacy messages that were not convincing enough. Advocacy messages may have been unconvincing because the messages lacked information or because the messages did not seem urgent, had little relevance, or did not employ appeal strategies. An advocacy team will need to revise advocacy messages so that the messages will be compelling enough to audiences that they take action.

Geographical or Demographical Differences

Geographical differences refer to the differences in the location in which various audiences are situated. Demographical differences refer to the differences in characteristics of audiences such as sex, age, race, and socioeconomic status. Geographical and demographical differences should be considered when correcting an advocacy strategy and advocacy messages because these differences can significantly shape how advocacy messages are corrected.

Geographical differences should be considered because audiences in different locations may respond differently to the same advocacy messages. For example, if advocacy messages were disseminated throughout the state of Indiana, audiences in other cities may have responded better to advocacy messages than audiences in just the cities of Fort Wayne and Lafayette. If such geographical differences in message receptivity occurred, an advocacy team should brainstorm why those differences occurred. For example, the differences may have been because audiences in other cities watch more news than audiences in Fort Wayne and Lafayette. If that was the case, an advocacy team could use another channel besides news for the dissemination of advocacy messages in Fort Wayne and Lafayette for future advocacy efforts.

Geographical differences in message receptivity also may indicate that advocacy efforts in certain locations were more successful than efforts in other locations. For example, if members of an advocacy team were split into three groups and each group advocated in the Indiana cities of Indianapolis, Fort Wayne, and Lafayette respectively, a lack of favorable responses in Fort Wayne and Lafayette may reflect how those groups responsible for advocating in those areas were not as effective in advocacy. If that was the case, the more successful group (i.e., the group in Indianapolis) should share the strategies that were effective for them with the other two advocacy groups. For example, the more successful group may have been less aggressive in putting the point across and more focused on building rapport with audiences.

Geographical differences in receptivity to advocacy messages also may have arisen if an advocacy team did not understand target audiences well. For example, audiences in Indianapolis may have responded better to advocacy messages disseminated online because they use the Internet more frequently than audiences in Fort Wayne and Lafayette. Or, it could have been that audiences in Indianapolis had more Internet access than audiences in Fort Wayne and Lafayette. In either case, such differences may have been mitigated if an advocacy team understood target audiences better.

Demographical differences also should be considered because audiences of certain demographics may have been more receptive to advocacy messages than audiences of other demographics. An advocacy team needs to ascertain why those differences occurred. There can be several demographical differences, including differences in sex, age, race, and socioeconomic status.

Demographical differences in sex may have been a reason for differences in message receptivity. For example, female audiences may have been more receptive to advocacy messages related to cancer than male audiences. This may have occurred because male audiences may have had a lower perceived risk of cancer. An advocacy team could consider expanding the scope of the revised advocacy messages so that male audiences may perceive risk as well. However, this depends on what the advocacy goal was. For instance, if the advocacy goal pertained to cancer in general, an advocacy team may expand the scope of the revised advocacy messages. If the advocacy goal pertained to cancer predominantly diagnosed in women, the advocacy team may not want to alter the scope of the revised advocacy messages. Differences in message receptivity also may have been due to different media preferences between male and female audiences. For example, male audiences may have preferred the television for news, whereas female audiences may have preferred the Internet for news. Consequently, more female audiences than male audiences may have received advocacy messages that were disseminated through the Internet. Again, depending on the advocacy goal, an advocacy team may consider using other channels for message dissemination or continue with the channel that was used previously. If the advocacy goal pertained more to females, the advocacy team should retain the use of the Internet as a channel for message dissemination. If the advocacy goal had a more general scope, the advocacy team should consider another channel that would communicate both to male and female audiences.

Age is another demographic difference that could have had significantly affected receptivity to advocacy messages. For example, younger audiences may have been receptive toward calls to support an advocacy campaign via the Internet, but older audiences may not have been as enthusiastic about the approach (see Xie & Jaeger, 2008). Also, certain appeal strategies may have worked for younger audiences, but less so for older audiences. For example, younger audiences may have been more receptive than older audiences to stimulating elements in advocacy messages, such as loud sounds and dramatic depictions. An advocacy team should revise advocacy messages so that age differences would not be an issue. An advocacy team could revise advocacy messages so that the messages would be suitable for older audiences and then disseminate these messages to the older audiences (i.e., separately from messages disseminated to younger audiences).

Differences in race or ethnicity may have been a reason for differences in message receptivity in audiences. As mentioned in Chapter 6, health information that integrates relevant cultural elements may better capture the attention of audiences and help stimulate information processing in those audiences (Kreuter & Haughton, 2006). In contrast, advocacy messages that incorporate culture that is not relatable to some audiences likely will not be well-received. Such issues could have been mitigated if an advocacy team better understood the demographics of target audiences. If race or ethnic differences in message receptivity occurred, an advocacy team should revise advocacy messages so that audiences of other races or ethnicities may relate to the revised messages as well.

Socioeconomic differences may have been a reason for differences in message receptivity. For instance, audiences who live in rural areas may not have had access to the Internet or may not have been familiar with using the Internet. Those audiences also may have lower literacy (see e.g., Ellis, 2007) and may not have understood instructions on the Internet. Such issues may have arisen if an advocacy team did not understand its target audiences well. An advocacy team should consider more suitable approaches for such audiences to support an advocacy campaign, such as non-Internet approaches to signing an online petition. For example, the advocacy team may set up a petition booth in the vicinity of the rural areas for those audiences to sign a petition on paper. Also, it may be beneficial for those audiences that the advocacy team is in the vicinity because the team may help elucidate concerns that audiences may have in regards to the campaign. An advocacy team will need to assess if socioeconomic differences resulted in differences in message receptivity and address those differences in the revised strategy and messages.

Geographical and demographical differences may have been reasons for differences in message receptivity in audiences. Geographical differences refer to differences in the location in which various audiences are situated, while demographical differences refer to the differences in characteristics of audiences, including sex, age, race, and socioeconomic status. An advocacy team should assess if there were geographical and demographical differences that affected receptivity to advocacy messages. An advocacy team will need to address those differences accordingly in the team's future advocacy strategy and messages.

Summary

If an advocacy team determined that the advocacy campaign was unsuccessful, they may decide to continue with the advocacy effort. The team will need to go through the Correction Loop before relaunching the advocacy effort. The Correction Loop is a phase during which an advocacy team cycles back to Phase 2 (i.e., formative research and message development) and Phase 3 (i.e., implementation and evaluation). The advocacy team will have to correct its strategy and advocacy messages based on the process and outcome evaluations. In particular, the advocacy team will need to assess the reasons for negative responses and geographical or demographical differences. Reasons for negative responses may include lack of information, participation apprehension, and unconvincing advocacy messages. Geographical differences refer to differences in the locations in which audiences are situated, while demographical differences refer to the differences in characteristics of audiences such as sex, age, race, and socioeconomic status. An advocacy team will need to assess what factors contributed to the negative or different responses toward the team's advocacy messages and address those factors accordingly in the revised strategy and advocacy messages.

The advocacy team will need to return back to Phase 2 and work on strategic planning, formative research, and message development based on those considerations. After developing the revised advocacy strategy and messages, the advocacy team will proceed to Phase 3 and implement and evaluate the strategy and messages once more. If the advocacy team determines the outcome of Phase 3 to be successful, the team may conclude the advocacy campaign by informing relevant populations about the health policy change or progress. If the advocacy team determines that the advocacy campaign was unsuccessful and decides to withdraw efforts, the team may conclude by informing relevant populations about the progress made. If the advocacy team determines that the advocacy campaign was unsuccessful and decides to continue the advocacy effort, the advocacy team will proceed to the Correction

Loop and revise the advocacy strategy and messages again. This cycle will continue until the advocacy team decides to conclude the advocacy effort.

References

Bandura, A. (1990). Perceived self-efficacy in the exercise of control over AIDS infection. *Evaluation and Program Planning, 13*(1), 9–17. doi: 10.1016/0149–7189(90)90004-G

Burch, E. E., & Henry, W. R. (1974). Opportunity and incremental cost: Attempt to define in systems terms: A comment. *Accounting Review, 49*(1), 118–123. Retrieved from http://aaahq.org/

Coulter, R., Cotte, J., & Moore, M. (1999). Believe it or not: Persuasion, manipulation and credibility of guilt appeals. *Advances in Consumer Research, 26*(1), 288–294. Retrieved from http://www.acrweb.org/

Ebbeling, C. B., Pawlak, D. B., & Ludwig, D. S. (2002). Childhood obesity: Public-health crisis, common sense cure. *The Lancet, 360*(9331), 473–482. doi: 10.1016/S0140–6736(02)09678–2

Ellis, C. (2007). Telling secrets, revealing lives: Relational ethics in research with intimate others. *Qualitative Inquiry, 13*(1), 3–29. doi: 10.1177/1077800406294947

Guttman, N., & Salmon, C. T. (2004). Guilt, fear, stigma and knowledge gaps: Ethical issues in public health communication interventions. *Bioethics, 18*(6), 531–552. doi:10.1111/j.1467–8519.2004.00415.x

Kreuter, M. W., & Haughton, L. T. (2006). Integrating culture into health information for African American women. *American Behavioral Scientist, 49*(6), 794–811. doi: 10.1177/0002764205283801

Kreuter, M. W., Lukwago, S. N., Bucholtz, D. C., Clark, E. M., & Sanders-Thompson, V. (2003). Achieving cultural appropriateness in health promotion programs: Targeted and tailored approaches. *Health Education & Behavior, 30*(2), 133–146. doi: 10.1177/1090198102251021

Moriarty, C. M., & Stryker, J. E. (2008). Prevention and screening efficacy messages in newspaper accounts of cancer. *Health Education Research, 23*(3), 487–498. doi: 10.1093/her/cyl163

Sedler, R. A. (2006). An essay on freedom of speech: The United States versus the rest of the world. *Michigan State Law Review, 377.*

Swinburn, B. A., Sacks, G., Hall, K. D., McPherson, K., Finegood, D. T., Moodie, M. L., & Gortmaker, S. L. (2011). The global obesity pandemic: Shaped by global drivers and local environments. *The Lancet, 378*(9793), 804–814. doi: 10.1016/S0140–6736(11)60813–1

Wallack, L., & Dorfman, L. (1996). Media advocacy: A strategy for advancing policy and promoting health. *Health Education & Behavior, 23*(3), 293–317. doi: 10.1177/109019819602300303

Witte, K. (1992). Putting the fear back into fear appeals: The extended parallel process model. *Communications Monographs, 59*(4), 329–349. doi: 10.1080/03637759209376276

Witte, K. (1994). Fear control and danger control: A test of the extended parallel process model (EPPM). *Communications Monographs, 61*(2), 113–134. doi: 10.1080/03637759409376328

Xie, B., & Jaeger, P. (2008). Older adults and political participation on the Internet: A cross-cultural comparison of the USA and China. *Journal of Cross-Cultural Gerontology, 23*(1), 1–15. doi: 10.1007/s10823–007–9050–6

· 1 0 ·

PATIENT ADVOCATES AND HEALTH ADVOCACY

Now that the Health Communication Advocacy Model has been thoroughly explicated, we shall apply the model in two unique situations. First, in this chapter, we will explore how one may advocate on the micro-level as a patient advocate. Second, we will explore how organizations advocate on the macro-level in the next chapter.

Traditionally, patients and their caregivers had a small role in diagnosis and treatment processes; physicians often regulated such responsibilities. Recently, however, scholars have advanced the concept of individuals stepping up to represent and help patients in the diagnosis and treatment processes. This concept is known as patient advocacy (see Kreps, 1996). In this chapter, we will define the concept of patient advocacy and discuss how health advocacy may be conducted at this micro-level. We will consider how one can begin by helping a patient and potentially progress to a full-scale advocacy campaign.

Patient Advocacy

The concept of patient advocacy refers to the action of representing a patient in addressing an issue (O'Hair et al., 2003). This concept is found both in the discipline of Communication and in nursing (see e.g., Baldwin, 2003; Bu & Jezewski, 2007). Despite differences in the definition across the two disciplines, it generally is agreed that patient advocacy involves championing a cause on behalf of a patient (see e.g., Bu & Jezewski, 2007). For example, if a cancer patient is constantly experiencing fatigue due to chemotherapy (see Goedendorp et al., 2012), a patient advocate may help represent the cancer patient by attending to time-consuming and often frustrating insurance matters. An advocate needs to understand the circumstances of the represented person and have regard and respect for the needs of the represented person (see Forster, 1998). Therefore, a patient advocate is not merely a distant bystander who comes along briefly to defend a patient; the patient advocate is an individual who thoroughly understands and empathizes with the experiences of a patient. Thus, the patient advocate usually is a patient's caregiver, but also may be a friend or committed volunteer, who is responsible for enhancing the welfare of a patient. A patient advocate also represents a patient in dealing with issues that may be challenging for the patient to handle, especially if a medical condition limits the patient's ability to address those issues. Thus, patient advocacy is similar to health advocacy in that an individual or a group of individuals represents another to address a health concern. However, there are subtle but important differences.

Health advocacy and patient advocacy differ in regards to the people represented in advocacy. Health advocacy can involve championing for people who may not necessarily be patients, whereas patient advocacy is exclusively focused on championing for patients. For example, health advocacy may involve representing a community in fighting against environmental pollution. In such a scenario, the community is not a patient or an individual, and therefore this type of advocacy cannot be described as patient advocacy. Although the differences are subtle, this clarification may help avoid potential confusion.

Health advocacy and patient advocacy also differ with regards to the end goal. Health advocacy, in the context of this book, refers to a movement that strives toward policy change. Patient advocacy, however, may not necessarily work toward policy change. For example, a patient advocate may simply ensure that the quality of interaction between the physician and patient is positive and effective. In such a scenario, there is no need to persuade a legislature to enact policy change.

Therefore, health advocacy may not necessarily be conducted by a patient advocate, and a patient advocate may not necessarily be conducting health advocacy. However, a patient advocate may choose to conduct health advocacy, during which the end goal of the advocate would be to persuade a legislature to change a health-related policy. Next we explore a micro-level scenario where one may conduct health advocacy as a patient advocate.

Health Advocacy as Patient Advocate

In comparison to an individual who has little interaction with patients, a patient advocate may better identify needs for health advocacy from observing the struggles that patients go through. Because a patient advocate would be regularly attending to the needs of a patient, the patient advocate likely would be familiar with issues that may burden the patient's health. For example, during the course of representing and supporting a patient, a patient advocate may realize that the patient's insurance is not accepted by certain hospitals. If the patient advocate considers this to be unfair, the advocate may consider conducting a health advocacy campaign to address the problem. Using this example, we will explore how the patient advocate can utilize the Health Communication Advocacy Model to address this problem with a legislature.

Phase 1: Assemble Team

Upon realizing that some hospitals do not accept a patient's health insurance, the patient advocate decides to conduct a health advocacy campaign in order to address this issue. Using the Health Communication Advocacy Model, the patient advocate embarks on the first phase—the Assemble Team Phase. The phase requires the patient advocate to convene a team, plan for fundraising if necessary, plan meetings and assign responsibilities, and to craft a position statement.

The patient advocate may initially find it challenging to convene a team. One question that the advocate may have is: "Where do I go to find the members for my team?" At first, the idea of recruiting health experts and community partners may seem a daunting task, but actually it is quite feasible. To start, the patient advocate may already have networks with health issue experts; for example, the physicians who attend to the advocate's patient are experts and may be willing to be involved as a team member. However, because physicians often are occupied with work, they may not be able to commit fully as a team member. If this is the case, the patient advocate may negotiate with the physicians regarding the role and responsibilities as a team member. For example, the patient advocate may ask that the physician only be involved in video testimonials that support the health advocacy campaign. This is just one example. Physicians may support the campaign in various ways, such as allowing the patient advocate to list them on the campaign website as physicians who are in favor of the campaign. By listing physicians as supporters, advocacy messages may be perceived as more credible (see Leuthesser, Kohli, & Harich, 1995). Besides physicians, the patient advocate also could recruit patients as the advocacy team's health experts. As mentioned in Chapter 3, patients, too, can be considered health experts because they experience firsthand the health condition. The patient advocate may enlist his/her patient as a health expert. If necessary, the patient advocate may recruit more patients and have multiple health experts. For example, the patient advocate may feel that having more health experts is necessary, as it may assist the advocacy team in appearing more credible. There are a number of ways that the patient advocate can find and recruit more patients, such as through networking in support groups or online health forums.

Community partners may include healthcare communities and coalitions. Because such community partners often are large in size, they should not be difficult to find; a simple search on the Internet should generate a few search results on relevant healthcare communities and coalitions. For example, there are many different kinds of cancer-related coalitions that one may find on the Internet, including Colorectal Cancer Coalition (Johnston, 2006) and the Breast and Cervical Cancer Coalition (Clark et al., 2009). The patient advocate also likely would have participated in one of these communities or coalitions during the course of supporting the patient. Similar to health experts, getting community partners to fully commit to a health advocacy campaign may be challenging. However, some community partners likely would be keen on and willing to assist the patient advocate in health advocacy. The community partners may play a role in several ways, including helping the patient advocate to network with relevant populations and disseminate advocacy messages to those populations.

A good avenue for the patient advocate to recruit public health and/or communication specialists is a local university. Sometimes, there may be professors who would be interested in participating in a health advocacy campaign. Again, professors also may be occupied with work and thus their role may be limited, such as in advising the campaign's strategy through phone or email. Besides professors, students with strong public health and/or communication training may be good volunteers to recruit; oftentimes, such students are ambitious, and they would volunteer for the effort to gain experience while doing good within the community.

The patient advocate may find a lobbyist through networks in support groups and community partners, or through a search on the Internet. Hiring a lobbyist usually is costly, so fundraising likely would be necessary. When the advocacy team is convened, the team would need to plan meetings and assign responsibilities. The team also would need to craft a position statement. In this example, the patient advocate likely would lead the team in crafting a position statement such as "all hospitals should accept all appropriate insurance without biases." When Phase 1 is completed, the patient advocate and the health advocacy team proceed to Phase 2.

Phase 2: Formative Research and Message Development

The patient advocate may identify target audiences through various networks such as from his/her patient's support group or from community partners (e.g., coalitions). The patient advocate likely would have had many existing networks with relevant populations because of the supportive role played for the patient. For example, the patient advocate likely would have attended several educational programs, healthcare organizations, and support groups, and formed multiple networks through these avenues. The lobbyist in the advocacy team can likely identify relevant legislators, and the team can determine the most relevant media outlets. After conducting research and gathering statistical evidence, the advocacy team may design advocacy messages. The patient advocate has an advantage during this phase; the patient advocate and the represented patient can be included as credible speakers for the campaign's testimonials, narratives, and/or videos. Thus, as credible speakers, the patient advocate and the patient can help add persuasiveness to advocacy messages (see Petty & Cacioppo, 1984).

Another advantage that the patient advocate has during this phase is that the patient advocate and the patient likely are able to accurately gauge how relevant populations would respond and thus design advocacy messages more effectively. The patient advocate and patient are able to accurately gauge responses because their experiences likely are similar to the experiences of relevant populations. For example, if the patient experienced insurance coverage problems, the patient advocate and patient likely will accurately anticipate how other patients with similar insurance problems may respond to the advocacy messages. After messages are developed and pre-tested, the health advocacy team proceeds to Phase 3.

Phase 3: Implementation and Evaluation

The patient advocate likely may have a preexisting network from support groups, healthcare organizations, or coalitions. This network may allow for easier and smoother dissemination of advocacy messages to relevant populations. For example, the patient advocate may liaison with his/her coalition to email advocacy messages to all members in the coalition. After the advocacy messages have been disseminated to legislators, relevant populations, and the media, the advocacy team will assess the outcome of their campaign. If the advocacy team determines that the campaign was successful, the team will proceed to inform affected populations regarding the progress or change in health policy. If the advocacy team determines that the campaign was unsuccessful, the team may decide to withdraw or proceed to the Correction Loop, during which the team cycles back through Phase 2 and Phase 3 with a reworked strategy and revised advocacy messages.

The Patient Advocate's Unique Role in Health Advocacy

Health advocacy campaigns may be initiated by almost any individual, including a healthcare professional, college student, volunteer, or a patient advocate. From the example above, we can see that a patient advocate is in a unique position to initiate health advocacy because of a patient advocate's level of involvement with the health issue. Specifically, a patient advocate is well-positioned to effectively conduct a health advocacy campaign because of his/her network and strong understanding of the advocated health issue.

Because a patient advocate is highly involved in assisting a patient, the patient advocate likely is acquainted with many relevant people in healthcare, including physicians, nurses, people from support groups, and people from healthcare organizations such as coalitions. A strong network may help expedite health advocacy processes. In other words, a patient advocate may already have leads when recruiting health experts or community partners for the advocacy team. For instance, a cancer patient advocate may ask the executive director of the local chapter of the American Cancer Association to serve as either a health issue expert or a community partner. The patient advocate likely would have participated in relevant health-related organizations, such as a coalition. Having already established a network with such organizations, the patient advocate may ask known individuals to collaborate or to be community partners with the advocacy team.

The patient advocate's network also may help expedite the needs assessment process. Recall that as noted in Chapter 4, an advocacy team should conduct a needs assessment to ascertain if an advocacy campaign is warranted and possible. The patient advocate's network may help provide the participants necessary for the focus groups, interviews, or surveys in community asset mapping. For instance, an individual who is not a patient advocate may need a source for participants, whereas a patient advocate only needs to ask people in the support group that the advocate and patient already participate in. Also, because of the patient advocate's network, finding and interviewing key informants may not be difficult. For example, the patient advocate may already personally know the manager of a local support community and can ask to interview the manager.

The patient advocate's network also may help expedite the message development process. For example, instead of sourcing for participants to pre-test draft advocacy messages, the patient advocate may contact known support groups to pre-test messages. Also, the dissemination of advocacy messages to relevant populations may be easier because the messages could be disseminated through the patient advocate's preexisting network.

A patient advocate also is well-positioned to effectively conduct a health advocacy campaign because of a strong understanding of the advocated health issue. This strong grasp of the health issue may help the patient advocate to more confidently lead the advocacy team. The patient advocate's knowledge of the health issue also may enhance the credibility of the advocacy team. The patient advocate also may help accurately gauge the effectiveness of draft health advocacy messages. As an individual personally involved with the advocated health issue, the patient advocate may be able to accurately anticipate how relevant populations may respond to the draft health advocacy messages. For example, if the patient advocate knows, through experience interacting with other patients and their advocates, that the biggest annoyance for relevant populations in regards to health insurance is the inflexibility of some hospitals in accepting certain health insurance plans, the patient advocate may recommend that "inflexibility" should be the major theme in advocacy messages.

Also, instead of finding and paying people to speak in testimonials, narratives, or/or videos, the patient advocate and the patient advocated for may be speakers in campaign testimonials, narratives, and/or videos. Not only will the patient advocate and the patient be credible speakers because of their experiences with the health issue, the advocacy team can avoid the effort and expense required in finding and paying others to be speakers.

Given these advantages associated with the patient advocate's network and strong understanding of the advocated health issue, the patient advocate is uniquely positioned to effectively conduct a health advocacy campaign. Table 10.1 presents an outline of the advantages a patient advocate has in conducting a health advocacy campaign.

Table 10.1: Advantages of a patient advocate.

Network	Knowledge of advocated health issue
• Recruitment of health experts and community partners • Recruitment for needs assessment • Recruitment for pre-testing • Expedite dissemination of advocacy messages	• Credibility • Gauge effectiveness of draft advocacy messages • Be speakers in advocacy campaign's testimonial narratives or videos

Summary

A patient advocate is an individual who represents a patient in addressing a health-related issue. Health advocacy campaigns may be initiated by almost any individual, including a healthcare professional, college student, volunteer, or a patient advocate. On the micro-level, health advocacy may work uniquely and differently depending on the person initiating the campaign and the composition of the advocacy team. In this chapter, we examined how one may initiate health advocacy as a patient advocate. We also highlighted how patient advocates are well-positioned for health advocacy because of their network and knowledge about the advocated health issue. In the next chapter, we consider health advocacy on the macro-level and introduce organizations that specialize in health advocacy.

References

Baldwin, M. A. (2003). Patient advocacy: A concept analysis. *Nursing Standard*, *17*(21), 33–39. doi: 10.7748/ns2003.02.17.21.33.c3338

Bu, X., & Jezewski, M. A. (2007). Developing a mid-range theory of patient advocacy through concept analysis. *Journal of Advanced Nursing*, *57*(1), 101–110. doi: 10.1111/j.1365-2648.2006.04096.x

Clark, C. R., Baril, N., Kunicki, M., Johnson, N., Soukup, J., Ferguson, K., & ... Bigby, J. (2009). Addressing social determinants of health to improve access to early breast cancer detection: Results of the Boston REACH 2010 Breast and Cervical Cancer Coalition women's health demonstration project. *Journal of Women's Health*, *18*(5), 677–690. doi:10.1089/jwh.2008.0972

Forster, R. (1998). Patient advocacy in psychiatry: The Austrian and the Dutch models. *International Social Work*, *41*(2), 155–167. doi: 10.1177/002087289804100204

Goedendorp, M. M., Andrykowski, M. A., Donovan, K. A., Jim, H. S., Phillips, K. M., Small, B. J., ... & Jacobsen, P. B. (2012). Prolonged impact of chemotherapy on fatigue in breast cancer survivors. *Cancer*, *118*(15), 3833–3841. doi: 10.1002/cncr.26226

Johnston, P. G. (2006). The Colorectal Cancer Coalition: Reflections on the future. *The Oncologist*, *11*(9), 970–972. doi: 10.1634/theoncologist.11-9-970

Kreps, G. L. (1996). Promoting a consumer orientation to health care and health promotion. *Journal of Health Psychology*, *1*(1), 41–48. doi: 10.1177/135910539600100104

Leuthesser, L., Kohli, C. S., & Harich, K. R. (1995). Brand equity: The halo effect measure. *European Journal of Marketing*, *29*(4), 57–66. doi: 10.1108/03090569510086657

O'Hair, D., Villagran, M. M., Wittenberg, E., Brown, K., Ferguson, M., Hall, H. T., & Doty, T. (2003). Cancer survivorship and agency model: Implications for patient choice, decision making, and influence. *Health Communication*, *15*(2), 193–202. doi: 10.1207/S15327027HC1502_7

Petty, R. E., & Cacioppo, J. T. (1984). The effects of involvement on responses to argument quantity and quality: Central and peripheral routes to persuasion. *Journal of Personality and Social Psychology*, *46*(1), 69–81. doi:10.1037/0022-3514.46.1.69

· 1 1 ·

ORGANIZATIONS AND HEALTH ADVOCACY

In Chapter 10, we explored how health advocacy may begin at the micro-level with a patient advocate. In this chapter, we examine health advocacy at the macro-level. Specifically, we consider several organizations that are advocates of various health issues. It should be noted that these organizations may sometimes "advocate" in the sense of representing others in supporting a health-related cause; these organizations may not necessarily conduct a health advocacy campaign to persuade policymakers. Nonetheless, their support is vital because it helps amplify the voices of those they represent. For example, if there is no large diabetic-care organization that supports diabetes-related research and monitors federal funding decisions for such research, policymakers may assume that there is no demand or pressure to fund such research and decide to cut funding for diabetes-related research. In this chapter, we list examples of organizations that advocate for specific health-related issues and discuss how such organizations may forward a health advocacy initiative.

Susan G. Komen

Susan G. Komen, commonly referred to as Komen, is a non-profit organization which exclusively focuses on fighting breast cancer. It was founded in 1982 and is widely known for its pink ribbon symbol. Since its inception, it has funded more than $847 million in research, and more than $1.8 billion in screening, education, treatment and psychosocial support (Susan G. Komen, n.d.-a). One of the main agendas for Komen is advocacy. Specifically, Komen strives to ensure breast cancer is a priority among policymakers and to enhance access to breast cancer care services. The following details the advocacy priorities of Komen for 2015 (Susan G. Komen, n.d.-b):

Support federal funding. One of the advocacy priorities of Komen is to ensure continued federal funding for breast cancer research and the National Breast and Cervical Cancer Early Detection Program (NBCCEDP). The NBCCEDP aims to help low-income, uninsured, and underinsured women in getting free or low-cost breast and cervical cancer screening and diagnostic services.

Reduce insurance barriers. Komen also advocates for policies to reduce insurance barriers. For example, Komen supports oral oncology parity. Currently, there is a disparity between insurance coverage for intravenously administered and orally administered drugs for cancer treatment; the burden of cost is much higher for orally administered drugs than for intravenously administered drugs.

Enhance access to diagnostic mammography. Diagnostic mammography is more costly than screening mammography because of the additional x-rays that are required. Unlike screening mammography, diagnostic mammography is not fully covered in Medicare, Medicaid, and most private health insurance plans. Consequently, diagnostic mammography can be a financial burden on individuals who need it and inaccessible for those who cannot afford it. Komen aims to evaluate policies to reduce or eliminate out-of-pocket costs for medically necessary diagnostic mammography.

The Amputee Coalition

The Amputee Coalition is a non-profit organization dedicated to supporting amputees and their caregivers, enhancing amputee patient care, and raising awareness regarding limb loss prevention. The organization started in 1986, and since then has developed into the leading national non-profit organization in limb loss education, support, and advocacy. The Amputee Coalition strives to raise awareness among those affected by limb loss regarding the coalition and its services, ensure quality care and support for amputees and their caregivers, provide meaningful services and programs for its members, and increase funding for the coalition's services (Amputee Coalition, n.d.-a). The following are some concerns that the Amputee Coalition advocates for:

Fair insurance access. Formerly known as the Prosthetic and Orthotic Parity Act, the Fair Insurance for Amputees Act looks to impact insurance policies so that coverage for prosthetic care will be equitable. For example, in New Jersey, the fair insurance law states that prosthetic coverage must be on par with other health services. Currently, not all states have passed the Fair Insurance for Amputees law. Some states that have passed the law include Colorado, Texas, Indiana, New Jersey, Iowa, and Illinois, to name a few (Amputee Coalition, n.d.-b). The Amputee Coalition continues to advance the Fair Insurance for Amputees Act and urges supporters to contact their legislators for support. The coalition aims to gain federal support from legislators and raise awareness regarding the challenges that amputees face so that the coalition may participate in a committee or subcommittee hearing to advance fair insurance coverage for amputees (Amputee Coalition, n.d.-c).

Action against disability discrimination. Some organizations or people may discriminate against people with disabilities (see Smith, 2007). For example, a company may decide not to hire a person because of his/her disability. To circumvent such discrimination, a civil rights law known as the Americans with Disabilities Act was passed, prohibiting discrimination because of disability (Amputee Coalition, n.d.-c). However, there may be organizations or people who violate this law and still discriminate against people with disabilities (see Gostin, Feldblum, & Webber, 1999). The Amputee Coalition works to protect members of the limb loss community from such discrimination.

Travel protection. For amputees, travelling via airplane may be met with obstacles at security checkpoints. For example, security officers may screen an amputee in a way that might be inconvenient and challenging for amputees. To circumvent such obstacles, the Amputee Coalition works with the Transportation Security Administration (TSA) to ensure reasonable and appropriate security screening for amputees. For example, security officers will not ask an amputee to remove a prosthetic device. If an amputee was treated inappropriately or disrespectfully during a security check, the amputee can contact the Amputee Coalition to open a dialogue with senior TSA officials to address the issue (Amputee Coalition, n.d.-d).

American Cancer Society

The American Cancer Society is a non-profit organization dedicated to addressing and fighting cancer. The organization was founded in 1913, and since then has been actively involved in cancer research and cancer education and prevention. For example, the organization has spent more than $4 billion since 1946 to find cures for cancer, including drugs to treat leukemia and advanced breast cancer. The American Cancer Society also has free community programs and services that help cancer patients with their fight against cancer. For example, there are free travel services for cancer patients who need a ride to get treatment and free lodging places for cancer patients whose treatment location is too far from home. Cancer patients also can participate in online I Can Cope classes to learn more about cancer or share experiences through the Cancer Survivors Network, which is a free online community for cancer patients and their families. One of the critical missions of the American Cancer Society is advocacy. The organization has a non-profit and non-partisan affiliate, the American Cancer Society Cancer Action Network (ACS CAN), which focuses on ensuring that policymakers position the fight against cancer as a top national priority (American Cancer Society, n.d.). The following are examples of some of the health advocacy campaigns that ACS CAN is advancing:

More funding for cancer research. ACS CAN and Stand Up To Cancer are collaborating on a project to persuade Congress to increase federal funding for medical research by $6 billion over two years, including $1 billion specifically for cancer research. This project is called One Degree, in which grassroots volunteers from ACS CAN and celebrity supporters in Stand Up To Cancer collectively put pressure on Congress to implement the requested funding (One Degree, n.d.).

Reducing and preventing tobacco use. ACS CAN has been actively involved in mitigating the use of tobacco. The organization works with state legislatures to boost funding for programs that provide prevention and cessation services. ACS CAN also works toward preventing children from starting tobacco use and helping adults quit tobacco use; the organization's proposed solution is to increase taxes on tobacco products. For example, the proposed "Tobacco Tax and Enforcement Reform Act," S. 826, would increase the federal cigarette excise tax by 94 cents, increase federal tax on all other tobacco products, and require better-enforced tobacco tax collection and crackdown on illegal tobacco activities. ACS CAN also strives to protect workers from secondhand smoke through smoke-free laws. For example, the New Orleans City Council recently voted unanimously against smoking in bars and casinos in New Orleans. Now, the bars and casinos in New Orleans are smoke-free, following in the footsteps of restaurants in New Orleans, which also are smoke-free (American Cancer Society Cancer Action Network, n.d.).

Organizations and Health Advocacy

Organizations such as those listed may sometimes "advocate" in the sense of representing others in supporting a health-related cause; such organizations may not necessarily conduct a health advocacy campaign to persuade policy-makers. In the event that such organizations decide to launch a health advocacy campaign, their advocacy effort likely will be formidable. Organizations are particularly well-positioned to forward a health advocacy initiative because they may have a large amount of resources. Having such resources gives organizations the advantage of being able to expedite advocacy processes, such as recruiting advocacy team members, developing messages, and disseminating messages. In this section, we outline how an organization would uniquely and advantageously progress through each phase of the Health Communication Advocacy Model.

Phase 1: Assemble Team

An advocacy organization likely would be able to convene an advocacy team with relative ease. An organization should be able to contact relevant individuals with its already existing network. For example, it is likely that a cancer coalition already would have health experts working or volunteering in the organization. If not, the cancer coalition could recruit health experts from its network of hospitals, healthcare communities, or community partners. Furthermore, a patient could take the role of a health expert as well, and thus there are plenty of prospective health experts within a cancer coalition.

An organization also should be able to easily recruit community partners. For example, a cancer coalition, by definition of being a coalition (Sabatier, 1988; see also Weible et al., 2011), would already have its own network of community partners. The cancer coalition would only need to contact these existing networks and ask if they would participate in the advocacy movement. If an organization does not already have a network of community partners, recruiting community partners should still be relatively straightforward because community partners likely would be attracted by the positive reputation and credibility of an organization due to its size and brand name.

In that same vein, an advocacy organization likely would be able to enlist the help of public health or communication specialists with relative ease because of its size and brand name. For example, it may be easier for a well-established organization to recruit public health or communication professors because the organization would appear more credible and legitimate. Also, an organization may already have its own public health or communication specialists working or volunteering in the organization. For example, an organization may already have employees or volunteers who are skilled in mass communication and are responsible for the organization's communication activities. Or, an organization already may have employees or volunteers who are skilled in and responsible for disseminating health information to the public. Such members of an organization may be recruited as the advocacy team's public health or communication specialists.

Although it is unlikely for an organization to already have its own lobbyist (unless the organization was a lobbying firm), it still is relatively straightforward for an organization to recruit a lobbyist. An organization could use its financial resources, where appropriate, to hire a lobbyist. Unlike an individual or small group of individuals, an organization should be more financially capable to hire a lobbyist. Furthermore, an organization could delegate the recruitment of a lobbyist to the human resources department, in which employees are specialists in recruitment processes.

Phase 2: Formative Research and Message Development

If an organization is healthcare-related, the organization likely will be able to identify and contact its relevant populations relatively easily. For example, members of a cancer coalition could be the relevant population for the coalition's advocacy campaign. If an organization is media-related, the organization itself can serve as the media conduit by which advocacy messages are distributed to the public. For example, if the organization is a newspaper company, the organization would not need to design and disseminate advocacy messages to another media outlet; the organization itself could disseminate advocacy messages through its newspapers. If an organization is neither healthcare nor media-related, the organization should still be able to identify target audiences without much difficulty. Given the number of workers in an organization, there would be ample number of people to carry out the task of identifying target audiences. In that vein, formative research and statistical data collection could be delegated to relevant and skilled individuals who already work or volunteer in the organization. For example, if an organization has student interns working for the organization, those student interns may be given the task of conducting formative research and collecting statistical data.

An organization may be able to expedite the messaging development process. If an organization has a department specializing in designing messages, such as a mass communication or public relations department, that department may be given the responsibility of crafting advocacy messages. Of course, someone who is a member of the advocacy team and is familiar with the vision and objectives of the team should supervise the crafting of advocacy messages. If an organization's services are congruent with the advocated health issue, the organization may use its brand name for building credibility of advocacy messages. For example, if an organization is well-known for its fight against cancer, including the organization's brand name in advocacy messages may enhance the credibility and legitimacy of those messages. Furthermore, an organization may include healthcare professionals who work for the organization in advocacy testimonial messages. The inclusion of such healthcare professionals may enhance credibility of advocacy messages that address a health issue (see Leuthesser, Kohli, & Harich, 1995).

Pre-testing of draft advocacy messages should be straightforward if the customers/members of an organization are affected by the advocated health issue. For example, a cancer coalition could recruit members who are cancer patients to participate in pre-testing of advocacy messages. If an organization is not health-related, it could use its financial resources to provide individuals with incentives to motivate participation in pre-testing advocacy messages.

Phase 3: Implementation and Evaluation

Dissemination of advocacy messages likely will be relatively easy for an organization with relevant networks. For example, a cancer coalition could disseminate its advocacy messages through its own network of support groups, community partners, and healthcare organizations. Whether the organization meets its objective or decides to withdraw from its advocacy campaign, the organization could inform relevant populations about the advocacy progress through those same networks.

Summary

In this chapter, we considered examples of organizations that advocate for specific health-related issues. The examples we summarized were Susan G. Komen, the Amputee Coalition, and the American Cancer Society. These organizations advocate for different health issues that are congruent with their health-related focus; for example, the Amputee Coalition advocates for fair insurance for amputees so that coverage for prosthetic care will be equitable, while ACS CAN advocates for smoke-free workplaces. Organizations are particularly well-positioned to engage in health advocacy efforts because of their pooled resources. These resources provide the advantage of being able to expedite advocacy processes, such as recruiting advocacy team members, developing messages, and disseminating messages.

References

American Cancer Society (n.d.). About us. Retrieved from http://www.cancer.org/aboutus/index

American Cancer Society Cancer Action Network (n.d.). Reducing and preventing tobacco use. Retrieved from http://acscan.org/tobacco/

Amputee Coalition (n.d.-a). About us. Retrieved from http://www.amputee-coalition.org/about-us/

Amputee Coalition (n.d.-b). My state has fair insurance for amputees, now what? Retrieved from http://www.amputee-coalition.org/advocacy-awareness/documents/what-does-the-law-mean-for-me.pdf

Amputee Coalition (n.d.-c). Federal issues. Retrieved from http://www.amputee-coalition.org/advocacy-awareness/federal-issues/

Amputee Coalition (n.d.-d). Travel questions/concerns. Retrieved from http://www.amputee-coalition.org/advocacy-awareness/travel-questions-concerns/

Gostin, L. O., Feldblum, C., & Webber, D. W. (1999). Disability discrimination in America: HIV/AIDS and other health conditions. JAMA: The Journal of the American Medical Association, 281(8), 745–752. doi: 10.1001/jama.281.8.745

Leuthesser, L., Kohli, C. S., & Harich, K. R. (1995). Brand equity: The halo effect measure. European Journal of Marketing, 29(4), 57–66. doi: 10.1108/03090569510086657

One Degree (n.d.). Here's why this matters, and how you can help. Retrieved from http://action.acscan.org/site/PageNavigator/OneDegree_Microsite_AboutUs_Page.html

Sabatier, P. A. (1988). An advocacy coalition framework of policy change and the role of policy-oriented learning therein. Policy Sciences, 21(2–3), 129–168. doi: 10.1007/BF00136406

Smith, D. L. (2007). The relationship of type of disability and employment status in the United States from the Behaviorial Risk Factor Surveillance System. *The Journal of Rehabilitation*, 73(2), 32–40.

Susan G. Komen (n.d.-a). About us. Retrieved from http://ww5.komen.org/AboutUs/AboutUs.html

Susan G. Komen (n.d.-b). 2015 advocacy priorities. Retrieved from http://ww5.komen.org/2015-Advocacy-Priorities.aspx

Weible, C. M., Sabatier, P. A., Jenkins-Smith, H. C., Nohrstedt, D., Henry, A., & deLeon, P. (2011). A quarter century of the advocacy coalition framework: An introduction to the special issue. *Policy Studies Journal*, 39(3), 349–360. doi:10.1111/j.1541–0072.2011.00412.x

· 1 2 ·

CONCLUSION

This final chapter concludes the book by recapping the Health Communication Advocacy Model. Although at this stage you already should be familiar with the model, this chapter can help reinforce key concepts learned. This chapter also provides health issue examples that you may consider when advocating for health issues in the future.

Review of Health Communication Advocacy Model

We defined health advocacy as the attempted effort to change health policies so that better health outcomes may result. The Health Communication Advocacy Model was then introduced as a tool that can be used to navigate through an advocacy process. Although there are other books that consider the topic of advocacy (e.g., Daly, 2011), this book is unique in that it focuses on the communication aspects of advocacy and centralizes communication as the key determinant for advocacy success. The Health Communication Advocacy Model is consistent with systems theory and is comprised of the Assemble Team Phase, the Formative Research and Message Development Phase, Implementation and Evaluation Phase, and Correction Loop.

Systems Theory

Systems theory helps describe and explain how systems operate. The theory suggests that a system should be open in order to survive (Miller, 2012). The Health Communication Advocacy Model adopts characteristics of an open system; its components are permeable and include interdependent subsystems and supersystems. This permeability allows the model to take into account environmental factors or situational changes and to adapt accordingly. For example, if the advocacy team runs out of financial resources, the model allows the team to revise its strategy and to opt against hiring a lobbyist.

Due to the permeability of the system, the environment influences and shapes the processes of the model, including input, throughput, and output processes. In the context of the Health Communication Advocacy Model, the input involves information regarding the advocated health issue and the output is the advocacy outcome. The throughput involves corrective or growth feedback that is vital for development and dissemination of advocacy messages. Corrective feedback involves monitoring for deviations from the intended goal and addressing those deviations so the system can maintain progress. Growth feedback involves changing a system so that the system may be improved. Figure 12.1 provides a graphical illustration of these processes.

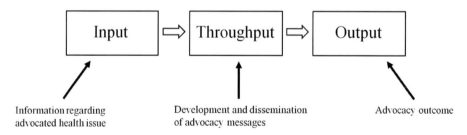

Figure 12.1: System processes shaping the Health Communication Advocacy Model.

From the above system characteristics, four properties can be inferred regarding open systems. These properties are: holism, equifinality, negative entropy, and requisite variety. A holistic system is a system in which the sum of the system's parts functions better than the parts working individually. Equifinality means that that there are multiple ways to reach the same goal. Negative entropy refers to a system's ability to survive and be effective. Requisite variety refers to the assumption that the processes within a system need to be as complex as the system's environment in order to effectively react to that environment. The Health Communication Advocacy Model is an open system and shares the above characteristics and properties. Figure 12.2 illustrates the Health Communication Advocacy Model and Appendix A provides a checklist to ensure all aspects of the model are followed for health advocacy. The Health Communication Advocacy model has several components, the first component is the Assemble Team Phase.

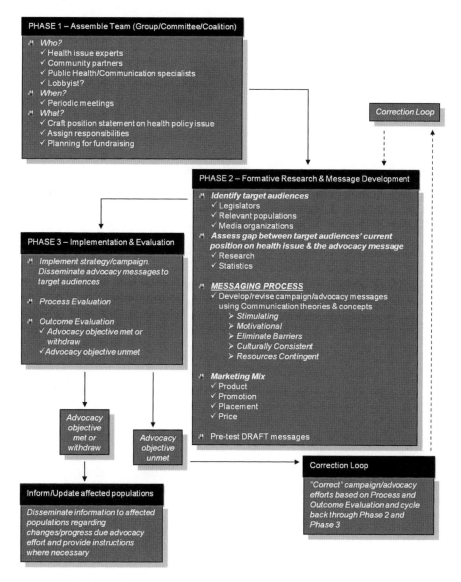

Figure 12.2: Health Communication Advocacy Model.

Phase 1: Assemble Team Phase

The first step in advocacy is assembling the advocacy team, which includes health issue experts, community partners, public health and communication specialists, and a lobbyist. Health issue experts are professionals with specialized knowledge in a particular health area. Health issue experts can contribute to the advocacy team by instilling credibility to the team and by helping the team avoid making medical-related mistakes. Community partners are grassroots groups and organizations that engage with the local community and may include unions, clubs, associations, health departments, clinics, universities, and so on (see e.g., Krieger et al., 2002). Community partners may help an advocacy team in acquiring resources, integrating new ideas, perspectives, and technologies, and providing a broader outlook of problems (Roberts-DeGennaro, 1987). Public health specialists are knowledgeable in disease prevention, public policy regarding health, and surveillance of community health (American Public Health Association, 2007). Communication specialists also may address health issues, but are focused on applying Communication theories and Communication research methodologies to health issues (e.g., Len-Ríos, 2012). A lobbyist is an individual appointed by a group to help facilitate in influencing public policy in the group's favor by contacting public officials, observing political and governmental movement, and advising on political strategies (Thomas & Hrebenar, 2009). A lobbyist plays a vital role in helping an advocacy team to navigate through intricate political systems. When an advocacy team is assembled, the team should decide on their position statement, which is the stance of the team regarding the advocated health issue as well as the goal of the team. The advocacy team should gather evidence pertaining to the health issue to develop persuasive and credible messages during Phase 2.

Needs Assessment

Before heading into Phase 2, the advocacy team should conduct a needs assessment in order to ascertain if an advocacy campaign is possible and warranted. There are three parts to a comprehensive needs assessment: SWOT analysis, community asset mapping, and key informant interviews. A SWOT analysis is a marketing tool that examines the internal and external attributes that can affect a campaign (Mattson & Hall, 2011). SWOT is an acronym that stands for Strengths, Weaknesses, Opportunities, and Threats. A SWOT analysis may help an advocacy team know the team's strengths and weaknesses and the environmental factors that may help or challenge the team and its efforts. Table 12.1 illustrates a SWOT analysis table.

Table 12.1: SWOT analysis table

	Helpful to achieving objective	Harmful to achieving objective
Internal Attributes (advocacy team)	Strengths **S**	Weaknesses **W**
External Attributes (environment)	Opportunities **O**	Threats **T**

Community asset mapping is a technique that involves mapping out the resources within a community (Griffin & Farris, 2010). Community asset mapping may help an advocacy team to determine what resources are available or lacking within a community and to plan the advocacy campaign accordingly. This technique also may help inform the team regarding the networks within a community and where the best locations are for advocating within a community. There are four ways to conduct community asset mapping: focus groups, interviews, surveys, and/or community walks (Healthy City, 2012).

Key informant interviews involve identifying and interviewing key individuals within a community (Marshall, 1996; Mattson & Hall, 2011). The responses of key informants may help an advocacy team determine if there is demand for health policy change. Also, the responses of key informants may be used as persuasive supporting evidence in advocacy messages. However, the opinions of key informants may not be congruent with the opinions of other members of the community (Marshall, 1996). Therefore, an advocacy team also should interview other members of a community.

After the needs assessment is completed and an advocacy effort is determined to be feasible and necessary, the advocacy team moves on to Phase 2: Formative Research and Message Development.

Phase 2: Formative Research

The first part of Phase 2 involves formative research. During this phase, an advocacy team will collect statistical and related evidence that will inform the team about the advocated health issue, including the prevalence, problems, and forecast of the health issue. The team also will determine its target audience in order to craft advocacy messages that are relevant and effective. Specifically, the team must ascertain what is appropriate, relevant, and important for its audiences, the audiences' level of awareness for the health issue, and how much the audiences know or do not know about the advocated health issue. There usually are three primary audiences for health advocacy campaigns: legislators, relevant populations, and the media. Legislators are politicians in charge of specific districts or states who are involved in creating and implementing policy (Bernheim, Rangel, & Rayo, 2006). Relevant populations are people affected directly or indirectly by the advocated health issue. The media are organizations that specialize in mass communication of information (e.g., news) through channels such as radio, television, newspapers, and the Internet. After an advocacy team gathers statistical evidence and identifies and understands its target audiences, the team will proceed to develop advocacy messages.

Phase 2: Message Development

The second part of Phase 2 involves message development. An advocacy team must aim to design messages that would persuade target audiences to be in favor of the team's position statement on a health issue. In order to craft such messages, five key elements should be incorporated: messages should be stimulating, motivational, eliminating barriers, culturally consistent, and within the resource capabilities of the organization or the advocacy team. A pre-test of draft messages should be conducted before messages are disseminated.

Messages can be stimulating by arousing the emotions of audiences (see e.g., Witte & Allen, 2000) and through the use of visual and audio techniques (see e.g., Bradley, Greenwald, Petry, & Lang, 1992; Bradley & Lang, 2000). Messages can be motivational by emphasizing audiences' susceptibility to a threat and how the threat affects them (see Witte, 1994), or by including self-disclosure in messages (see Han, 2009). Advocacy messages should eliminate barriers that may impede audiences from supporting the campaign effort. To accomplish this, the messages should anticipate and address possible internal or external barriers (see Allison, Dwyer, & Makin, 1999). Messages can be culturally consistent through "tailoring" (Hawkins, Kreuter, Resnicow, Fishbein, & Dijkstra, 2008) or through peripheral, evidential, linguistic, constituent-involving, and socio-cultural approaches (Kreuter, Lukwago, Bucholtz, Clark, & Sanders-Thompson, 2003). Lastly, the resource capabilities of an advocacy team should be taken into account when developing messages. These resources include time, money, and communication and organizational skills (Brady, Verba, & Schlozman, 1995).

Phase 2: Marketing Mix and Pre-Testing

In addition to incorporating the five key elements for message development, an advocacy team also should take into account principles of the marketing mix when developing messages. Marketing mix (Kotler & Zaltman, 1971) refers to the aspects of social marketing that are most important for achieving a successful social marketing endeavor. The marketing mix is comprised of: product, price, placement, and promotion.

Product refers to the recommended social action and how it is presented to target audiences. The product in health advocacy would be the notion of supporting the advocacy effort. Price is the cost incurred by the audience to engage in the social action, and includes psychological, monetary, energy, or opportunity costs. Place refers to the channel for audiences to translate motivation into action. The channel can be a physical location, such as a petition booth or rally site, or it could be nonphysical, such as the Internet or traditional media. Promotion is the act of bringing the product to the attention of audiences. An advocacy team may raise awareness of the advocacy effort through multiple approaches, including conducting a rally, using social media, or using traditional media.

After developing advocacy messages that incorporate the five key elements of message development and marketing mix concepts, the advocacy team should conduct focus groups (see Guest, Namey, & Mitchell, 2013) to pre-test those draft messages. Pre-testing messages can help rectify content and stylistic issues before actual dissemination of those messages. Pre-testing messages also helps an advocacy team to anticipate and prepare for the kind of responses target audiences may have. After pre-testing of messages is completed, the team proceeds to Phase 3: Implementation and Evaluation.

Phase 3: Implementation and Evaluation

Implementation of the advocacy team's strategy involves disseminating advocacy messages to target audiences. The approach to disseminating messages depends on who the target audiences are because the media, relevant populations, and legislators may each respond differently to those messages. The advocacy team will need to monitor the advocacy progress and evaluate the strategy and outcome. If the team determines that the campaign was successful, the team may conclude the campaign by informing relevant populations regarding the policy changes implemented or the progress that was achieved. If the campaign was deemed unsuccessful, the team may continue with its advocacy effort or withdraw from advocacy. If the team decides to withdraw from further advocacy efforts, it should inform relevant populations regarding any progress that was made. If the team decides to continue with its advocacy effort, the team should proceed through a Correction Loop and revise its strategy.

Correction Loop

The Correction Loop is a phase during which an advocacy team cycles back to Phase 2 (i.e., formative research and message development) and Phase 3 (i.e., implementation and evaluation). The advocacy team will have to correct its strategy and advocacy messages based on the process and outcome evaluations. The team will need to consider reasons for negative responses and geographical or demographical differences. Negative responses may have been due to a lack of information, participation apprehension, and/or advocacy messages not being convincing enough. Geographical differences should be considered because audiences in different locations may respond differently to the same advocacy messages. In a similar way, demographical differences also should be considered because audiences of certain demographics may have been more receptive to advocacy messages than audiences of other demographics. An advocacy team will need to ascertain why such differences occurred. After the team revises the advocacy strategy and messages, the team will implement its reworked strategy and messages and evaluate progress and outcome again. If the campaign results in another unsuccessful outcome, the team may choose to withdraw from advocacy or continue its efforts, during which the team will proceed through the Correction Loop again. This cycle will continue until the advocacy team decides to conclude the advocacy effort.

Health Issue Examples

Health advocacy efforts have been successful on numerous occasions. For example, the smoke-free airplanes we may take for granted today were a result of health advocacy campaigns dating back to 1969 (Holm & Davis, 2004). However, there still are many health issues to address; in fact, health issues are escalating (see e.g., Mariotto, Yabroff, Shao, Feuer, & Brown, 2011). Given the positive examples of health advocacy (see e.g., Freudenberg, Bradley, & Serrano, 2009), future advocacy efforts may help mitigate these escalating health issues. Although not meant to be exhaustive, the following are examples of health issues that may be addressed through health advocacy campaigns in the future:

Motorcycle Safety

According to the Centers for Disease Control and Prevention (CDC, n.d), there were 4,502 fatal motorcycle crashes in 2010. Fatal motorcycle crashes may be prevented if motorcyclists ride wearing helmets; helmets are estimated to reduce fatality in a motorcycle crash by 37 percent and the risk of head injury by 69 percent. Despite the effectiveness of helmets in saving lives, not every state in the U.S. has a mandatory helmet law, which requires all motorcycle drivers and passengers to wear helmets while riding a motorcycle. When a state repeals its universal helmet law, there is a sharp decline in the use of helmets and an increase in motorcycle deaths and injuries increases. For example, when Florida repealed the universal helmet law in 2000, the rate of helmet use dropped to approximately half of the rate of helmet use before repeal. Also, deaths of all motorcyclists in Florida increased approximately twofold, and motorcycle crash-related hospitalizations increased by more than 40 percent. The costs of treating head injuries due to motorcycle crashes escalated to $44 million after repeal. Given that helmets can prevent motorcycle deaths and injuries, it would seem very beneficial for states to adopt a universal helmet law. Since there are states that still have not enacted a universal helmet law or have repealed a universal helmet law, this is a concern that may merit consideration for health advocacy. Through advocating for policy change, a state may decide to adopt the universal helmet law and thereby prevent motorcycle deaths and injuries.

Health Inequity

Inequity refers to the potentially remediable differences between different groups of people (Starfield, 2011). Inequity may occur when people have similar needs but do not have similar access to resources, or when certain people have greater needs but are not given greater resources. Inequity is prevalent in the context of health too, and may occur between races (see e.g., Berry, Bloom, Foley, & Palfrey, 2010), gender (see e.g., Wells, Marphatia, Cole, & McCoy, 2012), and with groups that differ in income, education, or location, among others. Health inequity is a global problem; for example, an estimated 842 million individuals around the world are chronically hungry although global food production is sufficient to cover 120 percent of global dietary needs (Ottersen et al., 2014). Health inequity may be a product of social practices that are preventable. For example, within a university, the dining and food courts may not have many healthy salad options. In such a situation, students within that university likely have the same need for vegetable intake as compared to students at other universities, but they do not have the same access to adequate vegetable intake. A health advocacy effort may convince the university leadership to change university policy to implement healthy salad options within the dining and food courts. Besides advocating against health inequity in smaller communities such as in a university, one may consider advocating in other contexts such as inequity across cities, across states, or demographics.

Alcohol

Excessive alcohol consumption has been consistently associated with many problems, including lower GPAs (Porter & Pryor, 2007), impaired cognitive functioning (Mota et al., 2013), violence (Zhang, Wieczorek, & Welte, 1997), rape (McCauley, Calhoun, & Gidycz, 2010), and unintentional injury deaths (Hingson, Heeren, Winter, & Wechsler, 2005). Drinking alcohol in moderate amounts may circumvent such concerns; unfortunately many individuals consume excessive amounts of alcohol. Given the potential concerns that may arise with alcohol consumption within a university, such as rape (see e.g., McCauley et al., 2010) and violence (see e.g., Zhang et al., 1997), one may decide to advocate against alcohol purchase or forms of alcohol purchase within and around the campus perimeters.

Indeed, access to alcohol is increasingly easy for university students. For example, Palcohol can be purchased, carried around, and consumed at one's convenience. Palcohol is powder that, when mixed with water, becomes alcohol. In response to numerous problems that may be associated with Palcohol (e.g., spiking drinks and abuse by minors), the Indiana House's Public Policy Committee voted 13–0 in favor of banning Palcohol within Indiana. Other states, such as Utah, Tennessee, and New York may follow suit and ban Palcohol as well (Schroeder, 2015). Given that access to alcohol still is a problem in many universities, and given the problems associated with alcohol, access to alcohol is a concern that may merit consideration for health advocacy.

Conclusion

As health issues continue to escalate around the world (see e.g., Mariotto et al., 2011), the onus of responsibility is on people to make changes. Besides developing medicine and treatments to mitigate health issues, individuals also may contribute through health advocacy. Though there can be various approaches to advocacy, this book advanced an approach that emphasizes communication aspects in advocacy because communication is integral to persuading policymakers to implement policy changes. When you embark on your personal advocacy effort in the future, we hope the concepts in this book help propel your campaign toward success and change. In fact, this future may come sooner than you might expect. As you read these final words in this book, you have already taken the first steps into the advocacy frontier; you are now an individual well-equipped to initiate health advocacy through a communication approach.

References

Allison, K. R., Dwyer, J. J., & Makin, S. (1999). Self-efficacy and participation in vigorous physical activity by high school students. *Health Education & Behavior, 26*(1), 12–24. doi: 10.1177/109019819902600103

American Public Health Association (2007). *What is public health? Our commitment to safe, healthy communities.* Washington, DC: Author.

Bernheim, B. D., Rangel, A., & Rayo, L. (2006). The power of the last word in legislative policy making. *Econometrica, 74*(5), 1161–1190. doi: 10.1111/j.1468–0262.2006.00701.x

Berry, J. G., Bloom, S., Foley, S., & Palfrey, J. S. (2010). Health inequity in children and youth with chronic health conditions. *Pediatrics, 126*(Supplement 3), S111–S119. doi: 10.1542/peds. 2010–1466D

Bradley, M. M., Greenwald, M. K., Petry, M. C., & Lang, P. J. (1992). Remembering pictures: Pleasure and arousal in memory. *Journal of Experimental Psychology: Learning, Memory, and Cognition, 18*(2), 379–390. doi:10.1037/0278–7393.18.2.379

Bradley, M. M., & Lang, P. J. (2000). Affective reactions to acoustic stimuli. *Psychophysiology, 37*(2), 204–215. doi: 10.1111/1469–8986.3720204

Brady, H. E., Verba, S., & Schlozman, K. L. (1995). Beyond SES: A resource model of political participation. *The American Political Science Review, 89*(2), 271–294. Retrieved from http://www.apsanet.org/

Centers for Disease Control and Prevention. (n.d.). *Motorcycle safety: How to save lives and save money.* Atlanta, GA: Author. Retrieved from http://www.cdc.gov/

Daly, J. A. (2011). *Advocacy: Championing ideas and influencing others.* New Haven, CT: Yale University Press.

Freudenberg, N., Bradley, S. P., & Serrano, M. (2009). Public health campaigns to change industry practices that damage health: An analysis of 12 case studies. *Health Education & Behavior, 36*(2), 230–249. doi: 10.1177/1090198107301330

Griffin, D., & Farris, A. (2010). School counselors and collaboration: Finding resources through community asset mapping. *Professional School Counseling, 13*(5), 248–256. doi: 10.5330/PSC.n.2010–13.248

Guest, G., Namey, E. E., & Mitchell, M. L. (2013). *Collecting qualitative data: A field manual for applied research.* Thousand Oaks, CA: Sage.

Han, H. C. (2009). Does the content of political appeals matter in motivating participation? A field experiment on self-disclosure in political appeals. *Political Behavior, 31*(1), 103–116. doi: 10.1007/s11109–008–9066–9

Hawkins, R. P., Kreuter, M., Resnicow, K., Fishbein, M., & Dijkstra, A. (2008). Understanding tailoring in communicating about health. *Health Education Research, 23*(3), 454–466. doi: 10.1093/her/cyn004

Healthy City. (2012). *Participatory asset mapping: A community research lab toolkit.* Los Angeles, CA: Burns, J. C., Pudrzynska Paul, D., & Paz, S. R. Retrieved from http://www.healthycity.org/

Hingson, R., Heeren, T., Winter, M., & Wechsler, H. (2005). Magnitude of alcohol-related mortality and morbidity among US college students ages 18–24: Changes from 1998 to 2001. *Public Health, 26*, 259–279. doi: 10.1146/annurev.publhealth.26.021304.144652

Holm, A. L., & Davis, R. M. (2004). Clearing the airways: Advocacy and regulation for smoke-free airlines. *Tobacco Control, 13*(suppl 1), i30–i36. doi: 10.1136/tc.2003.005686

Kotler, P., & Zaltman, G. (1971). Social marketing: An approach to planned social change. *Journal of Marketing, 35*(3), 3–12. Retrieved from http://www.jstor.org/stable/1249783

Kreuter, M. W., Lukwago, S. N., Bucholtz, D. C., Clark, E. M., & Sanders-Thompson, V. (2003). Achieving cultural appropriateness in health promotion programs: Targeted and tailored approaches. *Health Education & Behavior, 30*(2), 133–146. doi: 10.1177/1090198102251021

Krieger, J., Allen, C., Cheadle, A., Ciske, S., Schier, J. K., Senturia, K., & Sullivan, M. (2002). Using community-based participatory research to address social determinants of health: Lessons learned from Seattle Partners for Healthy Communities. *Health Education & Behavior, 29*(3), 361–382. doi: 10.1177/109019810202900307

Len-Ríos, M. E. (2012). The potential for communication scholars to set priorities that curb health disparities. *Howard Journal of Communications, 23*(2), 111–118. doi: 10.1080/10646175.2012.667732

Mariotto, A. B., Yabroff, R. K., Shao, Y., Feuer, E. J., & Brown, M. L. (2011). Projections of the cost of cancer care in the United States: 2010–2020. *Journal of the National Cancer Institute, 103*(2), 117–28. doi: 10.1093/jnci/djq495

Marshall, M. N. (1996). The key informant technique. *Family Practice, 13*(1), 92–97. doi: 10.1093/fampra/13.1.92

Mattson, M., & Hall, J. G. (2011). *Health as communication nexus.* Dubuque, IA: Kendall Hunt.

McCauley, J. L., Calhoun, K. S., & Gidycz, C. A. (2010). Binge drinking and rape: A prospective examination of college women with a history of previous sexual victimization. *Journal of interpersonal violence, 25*(9), 1655–1668. doi: 10.1177/0886260509354580

Miller, K. (2012). *Organizational communication: Approaches and processes* (6th ed.). Boston, MA: Wadsworth, Cengage Learning.

Mota, N., Parada, M., Crego, A., Doallo, S., Caamaño-Isorna, F., Rodríguez Holguín, S., ... & Corral, M. (2013). Binge drinking trajectory and neuropsychological functioning among university students: A longitudinal study. *Drug and Alcohol Dependence, 133*(1), 108–114. doi: 10.1016/j.drugalcdep. 2013.05.024

Ottersen, O. P., Dasgupta, J., Blouin, C., Buss, P., Chongsuvivatwong, V., Frenk, J., ... & Scheel, I. B. (2014). The political origins of health inequity: Prospects for change. *The Lancet, 383*(9917), 630–667. doi: 10.1016/S0140–6736(13)62407–1

Porter, S. R., & Pryor, J. (2007). The effects of heavy episodic alcohol use on student engagement, academic performance, and time use. *Journal of College Student Development, 48*(4), 455–467. doi: 10.1353/csd.2007.0042

Roberts-DeGennaro, M. (1987). Patterns of exchange relationships in building a coalition. *Administration in Social Work, 11*(1), 59–67. doi: 10.1300/J147v11n01_06

Schroeder, L. (2015, March 18). *Indiana lawmakers move to ban powdered alcohol.* Retrieved from http://www.indystar.com/story/news/politics/2015/03/18/indiana-lawmakers-move-ban-powdered-alcohol/24969103/

Starfield, B. (2011). The hidden inequity in health care. *International Journal for Equity in Health, 10*(15), 1–3. doi: 10.1186/1475–9276–10–15

Thomas, C. S., Hrebenar, R. J. (2009). Comparing lobbying across liberal democracies: Problems, approaches and initial findings. *Journal of Comparative Politics, 2*(1), 131–142. Retrieved from http://www.jofcp.org/jcp/

Wells, J. C., Marphatia, A. A., Cole, T. J., & McCoy, D. (2012). Associations of economic and gender inequality with global obesity prevalence: Understanding the female excess. *Social Science & Medicine, 75*(3), 482–490. doi: 10.1016/j.socscimed.2012.03.029

Witte, K. (1994). Fear control and danger control: A test of the extended parallel process model (EPPM). *Communications Monographs, 61*(2), 113–134. doi: 10.1080/03637759409376328

Witte, K., & Allen, M. (2000). A meta-analysis of fear appeals: Implications for effective public health campaigns. *Health Education & Behavior, 27*(5), 591–615. doi: 10.1177/109019810002700506

Zhang, L., Wieczorek, W. F., & Welte, J. W. (1997). The nexus between alcohol and violent crime. *Alcoholism: Clinical and Experimental Research, 21*(7), 1264–1271. doi: 10.1111/j.1530–0277.1997.tb04447.x

APPENDIX

Checklist for Health Advocacy

Phase 1 – Assemble Team

Does the team have...

- Health issue experts? ☐
- Community partners? ☐
- Public Health/Communication specialists? ☐
- A lobbyist? ☐

When will the team meet periodically?

_____

Have responsibilities been assigned for each member? ☐

Have fundraising plans been determined? ☐

Position statement:

_____

Phase 2 – Formative Research & Message Development

Which approach did you use for needs assessment?

•SWOT analysis ☐

•Community asset mapping ☐

•Key informant interviews ☐

Have you gathered statistical & related evidence about the health issue? ☐

Have you identified these target audiences?

• Legislators ☐

• Relevant populations ☐

• Media organizations ☐

Did you incorporate the marketing mix?

• Product ☐

• Promotion ☐

• Placement ☐

• Price ☐

Did the advocacy messages utilize any of these key messaging elements?

• Stimulating ☐

• Motivational ☐

• Eliminate barriers ☐

• Culturally consistent ☐

• Resource contingent ☐

Pre-tested draft messages? ☐

Phase 3 – Implementation & Evaluation

Have you implemented advocacy strategy & disseminated advocacy messages? ☐

During this period, did you...

Evaluate process? ☐

Evaluate outcome? ☐

What was the outcome?

Correction Loop
Revise advocacy strategy and cycle back through Phase 2 & Phase 3

continue advocacy?

Advocacy objective met ☐

Advocacy objective unmet ☐

withdraw from advocacy?

Have you informed affected populations regarding changes/progress and provided instructions where necessary? ☐ (advocacy effort concludes here)

INDEX

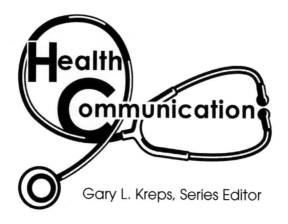

Gary L. Kreps, Series Editor

This series examines the powerful influences of human and mediated communication in delivering care and promoting health.

Books analyze the ways that strategic communication humanizes and increases access to quality care as well as examining the use of communication to encourage proactive health promotion. The books describe strategies for addressing major health issues, such as reducing health disparities, minimizing health risks, responding to health crises, encouraging early detection and care, facilitating informed health decisionmaking, promoting coordination within and across health teams, overcoming health literacy challenges, designing responsive health information technologies, and delivering sensitive end-of-life care.

All books in the series are grounded in broad evidence-based scholarship and are vivid, compelling, and accessible to broad audiences of scholars, students, professionals, and laypersons.

For additional information about this series or for the submission of manuscripts, please contact:

Gary L. Kreps
University Distinguished Professor and Chair, Department of Communication
Director, Center for Health and Risk Communication
George Mason University Science & Technology 2, Suite 230, MS 3D6
Fairfax, VA 22030-4444
gkreps@gmu.edu

To order other books in this series, please contact our Customer Service Department:

(800) 770-LANG (within the U.S.)
(212) 647-7706 (outside the U.S.)
(212) 647-7707 FAX

Or browse online by series:
www.peterlang.com